KT-116-990

Disclaimer

The information in this book is true and complete to the best of our knowledge. This book is intended only as an informative guide for those wishing to know more about health issues. The information in this book is not intended to replace the advice of a health care provider. The author and publisher disclaim any liability for the decisions you make based on the information contained in this book. The information provided herein should not be used during any medical emergency or for the diagnosis and treatment of any medical condition. In no way is this book intended to replace, countermand or conflict with the advice given to by your own health care provider. The information contained in this book is general and is offered with no guarantees on the part of the author or publisher. The author and publisher disclaim all liability in connection with the use of this book. The names and identifying details of people associated with events described in this book have been changed. Any similarity to actual persons is coincidental. Any duplication or distribution of information contained herein is strictly prohibited.

Hypothyroidism

And

Hashimoto's Thyroiditis

A
Groundbreaking, Scientific And Practical
Treatment Approach

Sarfraz Zaidi, MD

Hypothyroidism And Hashimoto's Thyroiditis :
A Groundbreaking, Scientific And Practical Treatment Approach

Second Edition, 2014

ISBN-13: 978-1490915968
ISBN-10: 1490915966
LCCN: 2014904102

iComet Press

6988 Calle Dia, Camarillo, CA 93012

http://www.icometpress.com

Printed in the United States of America.

CONTENTS

Section 2

TREATING HYPOTHYROIDISM AND CURING HASHIMOTO'S THYROIDITIS

PART TWO

RECIPES

Introduction

What is hypothyroidism? Quite simply, it means underactive thyroid. In other words, you do not have adequate amounts of thyroid hormone. Consequently, you develop symptoms of low thyroid hormone. These symptoms include fatigue, weight gain and thinning of hair.

You bring it up to your physician, who orders a blood test. Finally, you hear from your physician. "Well, your thyroid blood test is within the normal range. Therefore, you cannot be hypothyroid."

Sometimes, the blood test turns out to be abnormal. Then, your physician will diagnose you with hypothyroidism and as a knee jerk reflex, will place you on Levothyroxine, which is also called T4. Brand names for T4 include Synthroid, Levoxyl, Unithroid and Levothroid.

Despite taking your medicine, you often continue to suffer from symptoms of hypothyroidism or may even develop new symptoms. You discuss this with your physician, who runs another blood test for thyroid. Often, it is "within the normal range." Your physician reassures you that your thyroid level is "normal." Therefore, your symptoms cannot be due to hypothyroidism.

"But why am I having these symptoms?" you wonder. You may decide to seek an endocrine consultation or go online and try to find some answers. Often, you hop from your regular family physician to an endocrinologist to an alternative health practitioner, but continue to suffer from your symptoms.

The medical fact is that the thyroid gland produces two thyroid hormones, not one. In addition to T4, it also produces T3 (Triiodothyronine.)

Obviously, it makes sense to give both of these thyroid hormones, T4 as well as T3, to a hypothyroid patient. T3 is *extremely* important for our metabolism as well as for normal functioning of various organs in the body. That's why a hypothyroid patient on T4-alone therapy often continues to suffer from symptoms of hypothyroidism, such as fatigue, weight gain and thinning of hair.

Why are doctors so reluctant to prescribe T3? Because they have been taught to prescribe only T4 with the assumption that it will get converted into T3 in the body and everything will be fine. Often, they don't even bother to check the T3 level to see if their assumption is correct or not.

The medical fact is that T3 normally comes from **two** sources: It is produced directly by the thyroid gland. In addition, T3 comes from T4 to T3 conversion. In many individuals, this T4 to T3 conversion does not take place properly. Net result: you have low T3 and that's why you continue to suffer from symptoms of hypothyroidism.

Upon your insistence, your physician may *reluctantly* add a small dose of T3, which is usually *not* enough to provide you with the optimal level of T3. Therefore, you continue to suffer from symptoms of hypothyroidism until you find some physician who prescribes T3 and T4 in the correct ratio. Only then will your symptoms of hypothyroidism get better.

However, even this is still a *superficial* approach to treat your condition. Why? Because it does *not* treat the root cause of your hypothyroidism, which is Hashimoto's thyroiditis in a majority of hypothyroid patients.

Hashimoto's thyroiditis is an autoimmune dysfunction. In autoimmune dysfunction, your immune system goes haywire, seemingly becoming paranoid and mounting pre-emptive strikes against normal cells of the body, reacting as if they were dangerous and needed elimination. This is the basis of "autoimmune disorders."

For example, if your Immune System kills off your insulin producing cells (beta cells) in your pancreas, you develop Type 1 diabetes. If the target of the attack is your respiratory system, you develop asthma. If the target is nerve tissue, you develop Multiple Sclerosis (MS). If the target is the intestines, you develop Celiac disease, Crohn's disease or Ulcerative colitis. If the target is joints, you develop Rheumatoid arthritis or Systemic Lupus Erythematosus (SLE). If the target is the thyroid gland, you develop either Hashimoto's thyroiditis which often leads to hypothyroidism or Graves' disease, which often leads to hyperthyroidism.

It is important to realize that those patients with Graves' disease who receive treatment with radio-iodine or surgery continue to suffer from the autoimmune dysfunction, because these treatment modalities do not treat the autoimmune process in your body. Consequently, you remain at risk to develop any other manifestation of the autoimmune dysfunction.

What's the Answer? My Own Journey

In my early days as an endocrinologist, I too, used to treat every hypothyroid patient with Levothyroxine-only (T4-only) therapy, like most endocrinologists in this country and around the world.

Then, one day I read a research article in the February 11, 1999 issue of the *New England Journal of Medicine*, that would drastically change my treatment approach towards hypothyroid patients. The study compared the usual T4-only treatment approach to a treatment with the combination of T4 and T3. The results were astounding. Hypothyroid patients who were given a combination of T4 and T3 did much better compared to patients who were given T4-only therapy.

The results of this study made perfect sense to me. So, I started treating my hypothyroid patients with a combination of T4 and T3. Over the last fifteen years, I have seen some amazing results. Many patients who suffered from symptoms of hypothyroidism while on T4-only therapy simply blossomed when I switched them to a combination of T4 and T3.

However, this was only *half* of the solution. Despite a combination of T4 and T3 therapy, many of these patients would continue to suffer from autoimmune dysfunction. Sooner or later, some other manifestation of autoimmune dysfunction would *pop* up and we would go chasing it with full force.

My next step on this road was to see if I could get rid of autoimmune dysfunction at its roots. In this way, I could prevent my patients with Hashimoto's thyroiditis from developing hypothyroidism or other manifestations of autoimmune dysfunction. But how? The current medical consensus is that autoimmune dysfunction including Hashimoto's thyroiditis cannot be cured. You just have to learn to live with it. In fact, there is no treatment or cure for Hashimoto's thyroiditis at the present time. If you are diagnosed with Hashimoto's thyroiditis and have not yet developed hypothyroidism, the usual advice is to wait until you develop hypothyroidism. At that point, your physician will treat your hypothyroidism - often with a T4-only approach. A good analogy would be watching a train wreck in slow motion.

In order to cure Hashimoto's thyroiditis, we first need to find out what is its root cause. In medical literature, genetics is a well known factor that causes Hashimoto's thyroiditis or any other autoimmune disorder. Beyond that, medical literature is silent. With a fresh mind, I investigated what really causes Hashimoto's thyroiditis or any autoimmune disease, for that matter. I made some *amazing* discoveries. I was able to figure out the factors, (in addition to genetics), that cause Hashimoto's thyroiditis. All of these factors are related to our life-style and can be rectified.

Based on my findings, I developed a strategy to treat Hashimoto's thyroiditis and put it into practice. I am seeing some amazing results in my patients, many of whom are cured of Hashimoto's thyroiditis. In this book, I share this strategy with you.

Chapter **1**

Why Do I Feel Bad Despite A Normal Thyroid Blood Test?

A number of hypothyroid patients continue to suffer from symptoms attributable to hypothyroidism. Meanwhile, their physicians tell them, "Your thyroid test is normal. Therefore, your symptoms cannot be due to hypothyroidism." Patients feel annoyed and frustrated that their physician is not listening to them. On the other hand, physicians honestly believe that patients' symptoms are not due to hypothyroidism, because their blood test is within the normal range. This obviously leads to frustration, both for patients as well as their physicians.

Is it possible that you may actually be hypothyroid while your thyroid test is in the normal range? Let's take a closer at this question.

Blood Tests for Thyroid Function

1. TSH

Many physicians check TSH *only* to assess if your thyroid hormone level is normal or not. Why? Because this is what they have been taught to do. It is an *inexpensive* way to evaluate your thyroid hormone level, but it is not very scientific and often leads to an inaccurate assessment. So, if your TSH is in the *normal* range, your physician is *confident* that your thyroid hormone dose is good and your symptoms *cannot* be due to hypothyroidism.

In fact, this kind of assumption is *not* very scientific. It will become clear to you as I elaborate on this very common misconception.

Normal TSH Does NOT Always Mean Normal Thyroid Function.

TSH stands for Thyroid Stimulating Hormone. This is a hormone produced by the pituitary gland in response to the T3 level inside the pituitary gland. There is an *inverse* relationship between TSH and T3 level. Consequently, if your pituitary gland senses T3 to be low, it produces more TSH, which is a message for the thyroid gland to produce more thyroid hormone. Conversely, if T3 is high, then the pituitary gland produces less TSH, telling the thyroid gland to produce less thyroid hormone. In this way, the pituitary gland tries to regulate thyroid hormone production by the thyroid gland.

Often, patients *mistakenly* think TSH is their thyroid hormone. So, when they see low TSH on their Lab report, they think their thyroid hormone is low. In fact, their thyroid hormone may be high.

The Normal Range Of TSH Is Inaccurate

The so-called normal range of TSH is 0.4 - 4.50 mIU/L, which is **not** actually correct for many individuals. This range should be 0.3 - 2.0 mIU/L, a fact most endocrinologists know. However, laboratories continue to stick to the range of 0.4 - 4.50 mIU/L. Not too long ago, laboratories used to give a normal range as 0.4 - 5.50 mIU/L. It took them many years to bring the upper limit down from 5.50 to 4.50. It may take another decade before they bring the upper limit down to 2.0. In the meantime, you don't have to suffer from the *stubborn* attitude of the laboratories. Remember, normal range of TSH is 0.3 - 2.0 mIU/L.

Therefore, if your TSH is 3.8 mIU/L, your physician may be *erroneously* confident that your thyroid hormone is fine, but in fact, you may be low on thyroid hormone. In most of my patients, I aim for TSH to be below 2 mIU/L.

You also need to understand that a normal range simply refers to the general population. It is just a *guideline*, not an *absolute* fact for your body. For example, a TSH of 1.9 mIU/L may be normal for someone else in the general population, but not for you. Maybe a TSH level of 0.6 mIU/L is normal for you. Obviously, you will continue to suffer from symptoms of hypothyroidism at a TSH level of 1.9 mIU/L, even though it is in the normal range. In fact, your TSH needs to brought down further by increasing the dose of your thyroid pill. I have seen a dramatic improvement in some of my patients' symptoms, once I brought their TSH below 1 mIU/L.

Your TSH May Be In The Normal Range While You Are Actually Hypothyroid

Your TSH is a reflection of what is going on in your pituitary gland, not necessarily what is happening in the rest of your body, such as your muscles, skin, fat, liver, kidneys and heart. Therefore, your pituitary may be normal, but *not* the rest of the body, as far as the thyroid hormones are concerned. I elaborate in detail on this in Chapter 4.

In addition, there are a number of conditions which *prevent* the usual rise in TSH due to hypothyroidism. Consequently, your TSH may be within the normal range while your are actually suffering from hypothyroidism. More on this in Chapter 5.

TSH may also be *low* if your pituitary gland is *unable* to produce TSH to begin with. This happens in people who undergo surgery or radiation to the pituitary and hypothalamic area in the brain.

Sometimes, a large pituitary tumor or large doses of steroids may also cause TSH to be low. At times, the pituitary may undergo degeneration due to infections or acute hemorrhage, which causes TSH to be low.

Low TSH then leads to low thyroid hormone production by the thyroid gland. Your physician may *mistakenly* interpret low TSH as a sign of too much thyroid hormone (hyperthyroidism), and may inappropriately lower the dose of your thyroid pill.

If the cause of hypothyroidism is in your pituitary gland, we call it *secondary* hypothyroidism, as compared to *primary* hypothyroidism, when the cause is in your thyroid gland. We call it *tertiary* hypothyroidism if the cause is in your hypothalamus. It is only in primary hypothyroidism that your TSH may be high. However, your TSH is typically low or low normal if you have secondary or tertiary hypothyroidism.

2. Free T4

Free T4 stands for Free Thyroxine level in the blood. This is another fairly common blood test that many physicians order to evaluate the thyroid status of their patients.

<u>You May Be Hypothyroid Even When Your TSH and Free T4 Are In The Normal Range</u>

Let's say your physician checks your Free T4 in addition to TSH and both of these tests turn out to be normal. Now, your physician may be extra confident that your symptoms cannot be due to hypothyroidism. Really? A normal Free T4 does not always means your thyroid function is normal. Here is why:

Almost all T4 circulates in the blood bound to carrier proteins and is *inactive*. Only a tiny fraction (0.03%) of the total T4 circulates as unbound or Free T4. This Free T4 is *available* to tissues, but the Free T4 is still *not* active. It has to be converted to T3, which is the *active* thyroid hormone. Why? Because thyroid hormone has to bind to a *receptor* inside the nucleus of a cell in order to carry out its functions. This receptor is called the Thyroid Hormone Receptor (THR). Inside the cell, it is T3 and *not* T4 that binds to the THR. That's why T3 and *not* T4, is the true *active* thyroid hormone.

Therefore, your blood level of Free T3 (and not Free T4) reflects what is going on inside the tissues.

Most physicians treat their hypothyroid patients with T4-only therapy (Levothyroxine with brand names Synthroid, Levoxyl, Unithroid, etc). Why? Because this is what they have been trained to do. They have been told that T4 gets converted into T3. Therefore, T4-alone therapy should be adequate. Most physicians follow this recommendation without ever testing or questioning this myth.

In a scientific way, let's examine if the drum beat of T4-only therapy holds any water. Here are some basic facts in thyroidology that no knowledgeable endocrinologist would refute:

T3 in the blood comes from two sources: About 20% of it comes directly from the thyroid gland. The remaining 80% of T3 comes from T4 to T3 conversion. Obviously, if you are on T4-only therapy, your T3 level is 20% lower to begin with.

T4 to T3 conversion takes place due to an enzyme called 5' deiodinase, which is of two types: Type 1 and Type 2. Type 1 deiodinase is present in the peripheral tissues such as skin, muscles, bones, liver, kidneys and heart. Type 2 deiodinase is present inside the pituitary gland and the rest of the brain.

If your Type 1 deiodinase is *not* working normally, your T4 to T3 conversion will be inadequate. There are many *common* conditions that interfere with the normal functioning of Type 1 deiodinase, such as aging, diabetes, stress, surgery, infections, any chronic illness and certain drugs such as steroids. The net result? T3 in the tissues will be *low* and you will actually be hypothyroid even though your Free T4 may be normal.

Type 2 deiodinase present inside the pituitary gland is responsible for T4 to T3 conversion inside the pituitary gland. It is this intra-pituitary T3 that regulates the amount of TSH in a *reciprocal* fashion: low intra-pituitary T3 leads to high TSH and vice versa, high intra-pituitary T3 leads to low TSH.

Inside your pituitary gland, T4 to T3 conversion, carried out by Type 2 deiodinase usually stays normal. Therefore, your T3 inside the pituitary gland will be normal if your Free T4 in the blood is normal, as is the case when you are on adequate dose of T4-only therapy. With T3 in the pituitary being normal, your pituitary gland will *think* that your thyroid hormone is normal and will produce the normal amount of TSH. In this way, your TSH will be in the normal range, even though your T3 may be low in peripheral tissues (such as muscles, skin, bones, heart, liver and kidneys), and you are actually hypothyroid. However, your physician, in all honesty, will think your thyroid is perfectly normal because your Free T4 and TSH are normal. It is not your physician's fault. This is what they have been taught.

Another interesting observation: Your serum Free T4 abruptly rises by about 20% when you *fast* for 12 or more hours (1). In clinical practice, many patients actually fast for 12 or more hours because they also have their blood drawn for cholesterol, triglycerides and glucose level. This increase in Free T4 is *misleading* in the sense that it does not truly reflect what happens on a daily basis when you do not fast. You may actually be low in Free T4, but fasting will bring Free T4 in to the normal range. The reason for this abrupt increase in Free T4 after fasting is as follows: Fasting causes a decrease in the peripheral T4 to T3 conversion which causes a transient build-up of Free T4.

Therefore, next time you go for a fasting blood test which includes Free T4, do not fast more than 6 - 8 hours, which is actually enough for the measurements of your cholesterol, triglycerides and blood glucose as well.

3. Free T3

Free T3 stands for the level of Free T3 in your blood. Most T3 circulates in the blood, tightly bound to proteins. Only a tiny fraction, 0.3% of total T3, is present as Free T3. It is this free fraction that is *available* to tissues and is the active thyroid hormone.

Some conscientious physicians may even check your Free T3 in addition to Free T4 and TSH. When you are on T4-only therapy, typically your serum Free T4 level is in the upper half of the normal range (high normal), and your Free T3 is in the lower half of the normal range (low normal) for the two reasons I mentioned above: Lack of the 20% of T3 which normally comes directly from the thyroid, and inadequate T4 to T3 conversion in the peripheral tissues in a lot of individuals. Remember, your Free T3 and *not* Free T4 reflects your tissue level of thyroid hormone.

Case Study No: 1

An 80 year old Caucasian male had been under my care for his Type 1 diabetes. One day, he developed dizziness, for which he consulted his cardiologist, who put him on Microzide, a diuretic. His dizziness did not improve, so he stopped this medicine after about a month.

Then he consulted me for his dizziness. I ordered his thyroid function test, the results of which were as follows:

- **TSH** = 2.63 mIU/L (normal range, 0.40 - 4.50)
- **Free T4** = 1.1 ng/dL (normal range, 0.8 - 1.8)
- **Free T3** = 3.0 pg/mL (normal range, 2.3 - 4.2)

Clearly, his TSH, FreeT4 and Free T3 were in the normal range. Clinically, I diagnosed him with hypothyroidism. Dizziness is a common symptom of hypothyroidism, a fact many physicians don't know.

I placed him on Armour Thyroid 15 mg a day. Armour thyroid contains both T4 and T3. A week later, he called my office and was thrilled to report that his dizziness had completely resolved. Six months later, (at the time of writing this book), he continues to be free of dizziness. He wants to share his experience with other patients.

Case Study No: 2

A 72 year old Caucasian female consulted me for her hypothyroidism. She was having a lot of fatigue and dizziness.

She was diagnosed with Graves' disease in the past, for which she was given Radioactive iodine, which took care of her hyperthyroidism, but then she became hypothyroid, as is often the case. Subsequently, she was placed on Synthroid.

She was seeing an endocrinologist, who was treating her with Synthroid 150 mcg a day. On this dose, her laboratory values were as follows:

Free T4 = 1.5 ng/dL (normal range, 0.8 - 1.8)
Free T3 = 2.7 pg/mL (normal range, 2.3 - 4.2)
TSH = 0.85 mIU/L (normal range 0.40 - 4.50)

Although her TSH, Free T4 and Free T3 were in the normal range, she was experiencing severe fatigue and dizziness.

I switched her from Synthroid to Armour Thyroid 90 mg a day. Synthroid contains only T4 while Armour Thyroid contains both T4 and T3. When I saw her two months later in a follow up visit, her dizziness and fatigue had completely resolved. She felt like a new person. That's why she wanted to share this information with other patients who may be in the same boat.

On Armour Thyroid 90 mg a day, her laboratory values were as follows:

- **Free T4** = 1.2 ng/dL (normal range, 0.8 - 1.8)
- **Free T3** = 7.3 pg/ml (normal range, 2.3 - 4.2)
- **TSH** = 0.66 mIU/L (normal range, 0.40 - 4.50)

We can put these laboratory values in a Table form for an easy comparison.

Table 1

	Free T4	Free T3	TSH
Baseline (On Synthroid)	1.5 ng/dL	2.7 pg/mL	0.85 mlU/L
At 2 Months (On Armour Thyroid)	1.2 ng/dL	7.3 pg/mL	0.66 mlU/L

Lessons to Learn

The main difference between the two sets of Laboratory is the level of Free T3 which was in the low normal range when this patient was on Synthroid (T4-only therapy). It went up significantly, even above the upper limit of the normal range on Armour Thyroid (T4+T3 therapy). Her Free T4, which was in the upper normal range, came down, although still in the normal range. Look at her TSH, which stayed pretty much the same (and within the normal range) for two very different values of Free T3. It is pretty obvious that your TSH and Free T4 are poor indicators of what goes on in the body as far as hypothyroidism is concerned. In contrast, patients' symptoms of hypothyroidism go hand in hand with the level of Free T3.

This case also clearly demonstrates that your Free T3, Free T4 and TSH may all be in the normal range, but you may continue to experience symptoms of hypothyroidism if your Free T3 is in the low normal range.

****

I often see patients after their physicians, including endocrinologists, keep increasing their T4, hoping to ameliorate their symptoms. Typically, these patients have Free T4 close to an upper limit of the normal range (or even higher), Free T3 in the low to mid range and TSH is under 1 mIU/L and sometimes even below the normal range. At this point, physicians start to seriously doubt your symptoms are due to hypothyroidism, because they have gone to the extreme of fixing your hypothyroidism, but you still complain about symptoms. Only if these physicians knew this very basic fact: it is T3 and not T4, which is primarily the active thyroid hormone. Unfortunately, a patient will continue to suffer from hypothyroidism as long as their Free T3 is *not* optimal, no matter what their free T4 or TSH level is.

Remember, there is T4 to T3 conversion inside the pituitary gland due to **Type 2** Deiodinase which usually continues to function normally. It is this T3 level inside the pituitary gland (intra-pituitary) that determines the amount of TSH, in a reciprocal manner. A high intra-pituitary T3 leads to low TSH and a low intra-pituitary T3 leads to high TSH. A high Free T4 in the blood produces a high T3 inside the pituitary gland, which then produces a TSH which may be in the low normal range or even below the normal range. In this way, your high Free T4 and low TSH may *erroneously* indicate that you have a bit *too much* thyroid on board.

On the other hand, you may actually be relatively hypothyroid because of relatively low Free T3 in the peripheral tissues (such as muscles, skin, bones, heart, liver and kidneys), due to *impaired* T4 to T3 conversion due to a *decreased* functioning of **Type 1** Deiodinase.

In addition, these patients often become more anxious and may consequently start to have palpitations of the heart. Why? When T4 is high, it leads to high T3 concentration inside the brain due to *increased* T3 formation from T4 due to the normally functioning **Type 2** Deiodinase inside the brain. High T3 inside the brain can lead to anxiety, insomnia and palpitations.

Be Aware Of The Normal Range Of Free T3

The reference range of Free T3 reported by laboratories varies a lot. A free T3 level according to one reference range may be normal, but abnormal according to a different laboratory's reference range. A physician, who is in the tight grip of only looking at reference ranges, can be misled. Then, this doctor may make clinical decisions which may not be in the best interest of the patient. The reference range of Free T3 which I follow is 2.3 - 4.2 pg/mL or 230-420 pg/dL. This reference range comes from Quest Diagnostics, which is a highly reputable commercial laboratory, especially with respect to endocrine testing.

Remember, a reference range is simply a guideline, not a hard fact, for what is optimal for your body. For example, your Free T3 level of 3.1 pg/mL may not be optimal for you if you are still having symptoms of hypothyroidism. It may need to go higher, close to 4.2 pg/mL (or even higher) before your hypothyroidism is optimally treated, as is obvious from Case Study No. 2.

Your Thyroid Level Does Not Remain Static

Often, patients think that once their thyroid level is good, it will stay good. Think again! *The human body is not a robot.* Your thyroid level keeps *fluctuating* depending upon a number of factors, such as your weight, level of stress and eating habits, as well as any new medications or supplements.

Therefore, it is important to check your thyroid function approximately every three months, as well as when any new symptom of hypothyroidism develops.

Case Study No: 3

A 69 year old female consulted me for thyroid nodule and evaluation for Vitamin D. She was also experiencing excessive tiredness.

She was under the care of several physicians and was on a long list of medications, including Diovan, Keppra, Kapidex, Lipitor, Restoril, Gabapentin, Atenolol, Enablex, Zoloft, Xanax and Singulair. She was under a lot of stress at home.

On my evaluation, I diagnosed her with hypothyroidism. Her laboratory test showed:

- **Free T3** = 3.06 pg/mL
- **Free T4** = 1.0 ng/dL
- **TSH** = 4.78 mIU/L

I placed her on Armour Thyroid 30 mg a day. In addition, I also placed her on my Diet, which is basically a low carbohydrate-high protein diet. I also put her on Vitamin D3 as 10,000 IU a day.

At Six Months, she had lost 17 Lbs. Her laboratory test showed:

- **Free T3** = 3.5 pg/mL
- **Free T4**= 0.99 ng/dL
- **TSH** = 1.68 mIU/L

Her fatigue had improved significantly.

At Twenty Seven Months, she complained of excessive hair loss. Her laboratory test showed:

- **Free T3** = 2.26 pg/mL
- **Free T4** = 0.71 ng/dL
- **TSH** = 2.0 mIU/L
- **25 OH vitamin D** = 55 ng/mL

I assessed her excessive hair loss to be due to hypothyroidism, and increased her Armour Thyroid to 60 mg a day. Six months later, she was happy to report that not only her hair loss had stopped, but she was also growing new hair. She was feeling great. Her laboratory test showed:

- **Free T3**= 4.08 pg/mL
- **Free T4**= 0.79 ng/dL
- **TSH** = 0.13 mIU/L

Interestingly, her Free T3 was marked as *high* on her laboratory report, according to the reference range of 2.25 - 3.80 pg/mL, used by that laboratory. But according to Quest Diagnostics laboratory's reference range of 2.3 - 4.2 pg/ml, her level was in the normal range.

If I were to simply go with what the laboratory was telling me, I would have mistakenly decreased her dose of Armour Thyroid. However, I kept her on the same dose of Armour Thyroid. At the time of this writing she feels great, continues to grow hair on her scalp and is quite thrilled about it. She wants to share her experience with other hypothyroid patients.

****

4. Reverse T3 (rT3)

In addition to T3, T4 also gets converted into Reverse T3 (rT3), which is metabolically *inactive*. This conversion takes place under the guidance of an enzyme called **5** deiodinase (also called Type 3 deiodinase). Compare it to **5'** deiodinase (Type 1 and Type 2), which converts T4 into T3.

In healthy individuals, about 60% of T4 gets converted to T3 and the remaining 40% to Reverse T3.

Some health care providers like to do a blood test for rT3 in their patients. One has to remember, it is Free T3 that reflects the activity of thyroid hormone in the tissues. In this way, Free T3 (and not any other test) is the most *important* test for the true status of your thyroid hormone level.

5. Total T4, Total T3, T3 Resin-Uptake and Free Thyroxine Index

Tests for Free T3 and Free T4 became widely available in the past 10-15 years.

These advances have made a big difference in assessing thyroid hormone level more accurately. Previously, we used to rely on Total T4, Total T3, T3 resin-uptake and Free Thyroxine index.

Most T4 and T3 circulates in the blood, tightly bound to proteins, the most significant of which is called TBG (Thyroid Binding Globulin). The other two less significant binding proteins are TBPA (Thyroid Binding PreAlbumin) and albumin. *T4 and T3 in the bound form are metabolically inactive.*

Only a tiny fraction, 0.03% of total T4 and 0.3% of total T3, is present as Free T4 and Free T3 respectively. It is this free fraction that is *available* to tissues. Serum Total T4 and Total T3 tests measure your T4 and T3 bound as well as free fractions.

The main problem with serum total T4 and Total T3 tests arises because these tests are affected by the binding proteins levels. For example, if TBG is elevated, total T4 and total T3 are also elevated, and a physician may interpret that you have high thyroid level. But in fact, your Free T4 and Free T3 stay normal despite a high level of TBG. In the same way, if your TBG is low, your total T4 and total T3 will be low and your physician may inaccurately assess you to be having low thyroid hormone. But in fact, your Free T4 and Free T3 will be normal.

Conditions that cause elevated TBG:

- Estrogens in any form such as Birth Control pills, Estrogen replacement therapy, Estrogen-producing tumors. Even during pregnancy, there is high level of estrogens, which increases TBG level.
- Acute hepatitis
- Genetics
- Heroin and Methadone
- 5-Fluorouracil
- Perphenazine
- Clofibrate

Conditions that cause low TBG:

- Steroids
- Androgens, such as testosterone administration, DHEA supplements, testosterone-producing tumors.
- Nephrotic syndrome
- Cirrhosis of liver
- Genetics
- L-Asparaginase

In order to estimate Free T4, a special blood test was developed, called T3 resin-uptake, also simply referred to as T3 uptake. Make a note that this test does not measure T3 level, but T4 level. By multiplying total T4 with T3 resin-uptake value, Free Thyroxine Index is calculated.

Perhaps you can imagine the complexities we used to face in order to get an estimate of Free T4. Even worse, there was no easily available test for the assessment of Free T3. That's why most of the traditional knowledge focuses on T4 blood level.

With the easy availability of Free T4 and Free T3, the older tests of T4 really do not have any place in modern clinical practice. Surprisingly, a number of physicians continue to order these old tests, perhaps due to their old habits.

In Conclusion:

- T4-only therapy is the main reason why you continue to suffer from hypothyroidism.

- T3 and *not* T4 is the *active* thyroid hormone in the tissues.

- It is T3 and *not* T4 that *binds* to the Thyroid Hormone Receptor (THR), inside the nucleus of a cell, and carries out the action of the thyroid hormone. Therefore, inside the nucleus of a cell, all you see is T3 and *not* T4.

- T3 comes from two sources: directly from your thyroid gland as well as from T4 to T3 conversion in the tissues.

- Free T3 is the only blood test that *truly* reflects your thyroid hormone level in the tissues. That's why one has to focus on Free T3 level in order to diagnose as well as adequately treat hypothyroidism.

- Free T4 is *not* the active thyroid hormone at the tissue level, contrary to what most physicians *mistakenly* believe.

- T4 has to be converted to T3 in the tissues. In this way, T4 actually serves as a *substrate, a precursor* for T3, which is the *active* thyroid hormone.

- Free T4 reflects how much T4 is *available* as a substrate for T3 formation.

- TSH reflects whether the amount of T3 inside the pituitary gland is normal, low or high. It does not tell you what is going on inside the peripheral tissues such as skin, muscles, fat, bones, liver, heart and kidneys. In this way, TSH is a test for the health of the pituitary and *not* necessarily the health of the peripheral tissues.

- In clinical practice, both Free T4 and TSH are of some value, but these tests cannot replace **Free T3 as the single most important test** for evaluating your thyroid function.

- What laboratory reports as the Normal Ranges of Free T3 , Free T4 and TSH are simply a *reference* to the *young healthy* population. Your blood test may be within the normal range, but you may still be hypothyroid. In such a case, you may need to get your Free T3 close to the upper limit of the normal range, or even a little higher, to get rid of your symptoms of hypothyroidism.

- Different laboratories report different "Normal Ranges." The optimal normal ranges for the thyroid blood test are as follows:

Optimal Normal Ranges for Thyroid Lab Tests

Free T3	3.0 - 4.2 pg/ml
Free T4	0.7 - 1.4 ng/dl
TSH	0.3 - 2.0 mIU/L

Hypothyroidism May *Not* Be the Only Cause of Your Symptoms

You still may have symptoms, despite a perfectly normal Free T4, Free T3 and TSH. Now what? Your symptoms, such as fatigue, weight gain and thinning of hair are not limited to hypothyroidism. Many other common medical conditions can give rise to these symptoms and your physician should look into those. More on it in Chapter 3.

References

1. Nicoloff J, LoPresti J, Non-thyroidal illnesses.
Endocrinology/edited by Leslie DeGroot et al, Vol.1, 3rd edition.
W.B. Saunders Company, 1995.

Chapter 2

What are the Symptoms of Hypothyroidism?

Hypothyroidism is a state of decreased metabolism at the tissue level. In this way, every tissue in your body is functioning at a *suboptimal* level when you are hypothyroid.

The symptoms of hypothyroidism develop insidiously and are often non-specific in the early stages. Typically, a person may have symptoms of mild hypothyroidism for months or even years before a diagnosis of hypothyroidism is made.

The common symptoms of hypothyroidism are:

1. Weight gain (or difficulty losing weight), due to a number of factors including decreased metabolism and water-retention due to hypothyroidism. In addition, usually there is stress-eating behavior and decreased exercise due to weakness, depression, and muscle aches and pains. All of these factors add to your weight gain.

2. Fatigue, which is due to decreased metabolism, as well as other effects of hypothyroidism, such as depressed mood, weight gain, muscle aches and pains, anemia and decreased cardiac output (pumping action of heart).

In addition, there are other factors that can contribute to your fatigue. These are the conditions which occur more frequently in patients with Hashimoto's thyroiditis: Stress, Vitamin B12 deficiency, Type 1 diabetes, Adrenal Insufficiency and Rheumatologic Diseases.

3. Hair loss/thinning of hair, which affects the head as well as the rest of the body. In particular, there is thinning of hair at the outer side of the eye-brows. Nails are brittle and grow very slowly.

4. Decreased body temperature due to a decrease in the basal metabolic rate. Intolerance to cold temperature.

5. Skin is puffy, cool and dry. There is puffiness around the eyes, coarse facial features, swelling of hands and feet and supra-clavicular fossae (space above your collar bones). This is due to deposition of a *mucinous* (gelatin-like) substance in the subcutaneous tissues. Hence, it is also called myxedema. Swelling of hands and feet in hypothyroidism is non-pitting, which means the skin does *not* indent if you press it with your thumb. In comparison, swelling of the feet due to water-retention in heart failure is a pitting type (the skin does indent when pressed with your thumb).
Mucinous material can accumulate in other tissues as well, such as the heart, muscles and nerves.
The skin is dry due to a decrease in the function of sweat and sebaceous glands. The skin is cold due to poor circulation. The skin may look pale due to decreased blood circulation and anemia. In some patients, the skin may even get a yellowish tint due to accumulation of carotene in the blood, as its conversion to Vitamin A is decreased in hypothyroidism.

6. Muscle cramps, joint pains, accumulation of fluid in the Joints, known as effusions. Muscles are typically stiff and do not relax easily, which gives rise to muscle aches and pains. Stiff muscles also causes tendon reflexes (done by your physician) to be slowed, especially the relaxation phase, which is called "hung-up reflexes."

7. Constipation due to decreased intestinal movement. Sometimes, it can lead to gaseous distention of the intestines, called *myxedema ileus*. In extreme cases, fecal impaction can develop.

8. Atrophic gastritis is present in about 50% of hypothyroid patients. Atrophic gastritis is an autoimmune disorder of the stomach in which there is thinning of the lining of the stomach wall. This leads to a virtual absence of hydrochloric acid secretion by the stomach cells, which causes inability to digest food. In addition, the stomach lining is unable to produce a substance called Intrinsic Factor (IF), which is normally required for the absorption of Vitamin B12. Consequently, there is a lack of Vitamin B12 absorption, causing Vitamin B12 deficiency, with or without pernicious anemia

9. Depression, lethargy, lack of motivation.

10. Decrease in cognitive function, forgetfulness, and decreased memory. Some patients are mistakenly labeled as having Alzheimer's dementia.

11. Night blindness due to decrease in synthesis of *Retinal* from vitamin A.

12. Dizziness, due to malfunction of the inner ear and cerebellum.

13. Lack of balance, which happens due to accumulation of mucinous material in the cerebellum. Lack of balance may also be due to Vitamin B12 deficiency.

14. Compression of nerves, such as "Carpal tunnel syndrome," which causes tingling and numbness in the hands.

15. Slowing of heart rate, high diastolic blood pressure and swelling of feet. There is accumulation of mucinous material inside the muscle of the heart. Cardiac output (pumping of heart) is decreased. In addition, peripheral vascular resistance is increased, which causes poor circulation. There may also be pericardial effusion (fluid accumulation in the sac around the heart.) CK (Creatine Kinase) in the blood may be elevated. All of the above findings collectively are called *myxedema heart*.

16. High total cholesterol, high LDL cholesterol and high Triglycerides level.

17. Husky voice, enlarged tongue and sleep apnea.

18. Sometimes an enlarged thyroid gland (known as a goiter) is also present, especially in patients with Hashimoto's thyroiditis.

19. Pleural effusion (fluid accumulation in the sac around the lung) which is often small and does not cause any symptoms.

20. Menstrual irregularities, usually excessive and prolonged menstrual flow, giving rise to iron deficiency with or without anemia. However, sometimes, hypothyroidism is associated with an increase in Prolactin, a hormone produced by the Pituitary gland. High Prolactin level can cause lack of menses and milky discharge from the nipples. Prolactin can be easily measured in a fasting blood test.

21. Frequent miscarriages and decreased fertility. Decreased libido in both women and men.

22. In children, there is slowed growth and in young children, mental retardation when hypothyroidism is undiagnosed and untreated, which is also called cretinism. Untreated hypothyroidism is older children causes short stature and delayed puberty.

23. Prolonged, untreated hypothyroidism can lead to a coma, known as *myxedema coma*, which carries a high mortality if treatment is not initiated promptly. Certain factors can trigger *myxedema coma*, which include exposure to severe cold, trauma and infections.

Chapter 3

Hypothyroidism May Not Be the Only Cause of Your Symptoms

The symptoms of hypothyroidism are not limited to hypothyroidism. Many other medical conditions can give rise to these symptoms. Your physician may not investigate these medical conditions.

Instead, your doctor may keep increasing the dose of your thyroid hormone hoping to get rid of symptoms, such as weight gain and fatigue. Often, you end up on excessive doses of thyroid hormone and continue to suffer from weight gain and fatigue. Meanwhile, you and your physician blame all of your weight gain and fatigue on hypothyroidism.

Too much thyroid hormone often adds to anxiety and insomnia, both of which further worsen fatigue. Too much thyroid hormone also causes heart palpitations, tinnitus (ringing in the ears), and a decease in bone density, which leads to osteoporosis. For heart palpitations, physicians usually prescribe a beta-blocker drug, which further adds to fatigue.

To much thyroid hormone may lead to development of atrial fibrillation (marked irregularity of heart beat), which places patients at a high risk of a stroke. Can you see how trying to get more energy simply through larger doses of thyroid hormone can get you into real mess?

Weight Gain is often due to excessive eating behavior, aging and sedentary lifestyle. As we get older, especially over the age of 40, our metabolism slows down, but our eating habits do not change. Often, we also become sedentary due to one reason or another. In this way, excessive eating, aging and sedentary lifestyle play a major role in causing weight gain in people with and without hypothyroidism. Obviously, weight gain is worse if hypothyroidism is not correctly treated.

It is my clinical observation that obesity itself can cause hypothyroidism. Why? Because the thyroid gland has a limited capacity to produce thyroid hormone and thyroid hormone requirements of your body are weight dependent. The more you weigh, the more thyroid hormone you need. When the thyroid gland cannot produce enough thyroid hormone in proportion to your weight gain, you develop hypothyroidism.

Even if you go on a thyroid hormone pill that contains both T4 and T3, but do not change your eating behavior, you may not lose weight. Rather, you will have to keep increasing the dose of your thyroid pill to keep up with your weight gain.

You get trapped in a vicious cycle: Hypothyroidism causing weight gain, which itself worsens hypothyroidism, which causes more weight gain and the cycle continues.

Fatigue can be due to a number of factors, other than hypothyroidism. Physical, mental and emotional stress, sleep deprivation, obesity, sleep apnea, vitamin B12 deficiency, vitamin D deficiency, chronic low back pain, side-effects from medicines and post-meal reactive hypoglycemia are common causes of fatigue.

Stress not only causes fatigue directly, but also indirectly through a number of ways:

- Stress causes anxiety, insomnia and sleep deprivation, which gives rise to day-time somnolence and fatigue.

- Stress causes weight gain through stress-eating behavior, which leads to worsening of hypothyroidism. Weight gain itself causes fatigue, as you carry extra weight all day long.

- Stress also produces excess cortisol in your body. That's why cortisol is called the stress hormone. Excess cortisol has a *negative* effect on Type 1 deiodinase, the enzyme required to convert T4 into T3 in your tissues. In this way, you end up having Low T3 in your tissues which leads to fatigue.

- Stress also causes depression, which causes lack of motivation and fatigue. In addition, depressed people usually have a high level of cortisol, which inhibits Type 1 Deiodinase and consequently, decreased T3 production from T4, which leads to worsening of hypothyroidism.

- High cortisol due to stress has a negative effect on TSH production. This occurs due to the inhibitory effect of excess cortisol on the hypothalamus, which is an endocrine gland lying above the pituitary gland. The hypothalamus influences TSH production in the pituitary, by producing a hormone, called TRH (Thyrotropin Releasing Hormone). A high cortisol level inhibits TRH, which then inhibits TSH, which sends a message to the thyroid gland to produce less thyroid hormone, which causes fatigue.
In addition to excess cortisol, TRH secretion may be inhibited in depressed individuals because the hypothalamus lies next to the Limbic System, which is the brain center for emotions. The hypothalamus and limbic system are connected to each other through nerve fibers. In this way, negative emotions of depression can cause low TRH, which leads to low TSH production, and the end result is low thyroid hormone production and fatigue.

- Stress is one of the main reasons why people develop autoimmune dysfunction. Hashimoto's Thyroiditis is one of the manifestations of Autoimmune Dysfunction, which is a very common cause of hypothyroidism. Some of the other manifestations of Autoimmune Dysfunction that can cause fatigue include Vitamin B12 Deficiency, Celiac Disease, Adrenal Insufficiency (also known as Addison's Disease), Type 1 Diabetes, Rheumatoid Arthritis, Lupus and Fibromyalgia. When you have one manifestation of autoimmune dysfunction, you are prone to develop other manifestations as well.

- The association between Hashimoto's Thyroiditis and Addison's Disease is called Schmidt's Syndrome. Sometimes, Addison's disease becomes clinically apparent when a patient with hypothyroidism starts to take thyroid hormone. In Addison's disease, your cortisol production is very low. Therefore, instead of feeling better when taking thyroid hormone, you start to feel worse. In particular, there is worsening of fatigue to the point of severe exhaustion. If not promptly diagnosed and appropriately treated, a patient may end up having an Addisonian Crisis, which is a life-threatening condition. In Addisonian Crisis, you have very low blood pressure and abnormally elevated serum potassium level, both of which can rapidly lead to death if not treated promptly.

This is how the initiation of hypothyroidism treatment can precipitate an Addisonian Crisis. A patient with hypothyroidism may have adrenal insufficiency (Addison's disease) of a mild degree, with a low production of cortisol, but is not diagnosed with it yet. The initiation of thyroid hormone increases the breakdown of cortisol, which further decreases the already low serum cortisol level.

To diagnose Addison's disease, you need a special test called <u>ACTH stimulation test</u>. In this test, you have your blood drawn for serum cortisol before and 60 minutes after the injection of 250 micrograms of synthetic ACTH, called Cosyntropin (brand name Cortrosyn). You need a physician's order for this blood test.

Post-meal, reactive hypoglycemia occurs in people who have insulin resistance after they ingest refined sugars, such as juices. A sudden rise of glucose causes their pancreas to produce a large amount of insulin, which rapidly brings their blood glucose down. A sudden rise and sudden fall in blood glucose gives rise to symptoms of hypoglycemia, even though blood glucose may be in the normal range.

After a couple of hours, juice from the stomach is long gone, but there is still a large amount of insulin circulating in the blood. Consequently, blood glucose may get down into the low range, which causes severe fatigue and mental fogginess. Post-meal, reactive hypoglycemia can easily be diagnosed on a 2-hour Oral Glucose Tolerance Test.

Hair loss is often due to stress in addition to hypothyroidism. Stress can be physical, such as an illness, or psychological, such as anxiety. Hair loss can also be due to Vitamin B12 deficiency, iron deficiency, and side-effects from drugs. Some of the commonly used drugs that can cause hair loss include NSAIDS (Non-Steroidal Anti-inflammatory Drugs), antibiotics, antifungal drugs, anti-depressants, birth control pills, cholesterol lowering drugs, anti-clotting drugs, chemotherapy agents and anti-hypertensive drugs such as ACE-inhibitors and Beta-blockers.

Hair loss can also be due Alopecia areata, which is an autoimmune disorder. It occurs more frequently in patients with Hashimoto's thyroiditis, which is also an autoimmune disorder.

Hair loss itself triggers anxiety which plays a major role in causing Alopecia areata, Hashimoto's thyroiditis and hypothyroidism. In this way, a vicious cycle sets in.

Muscle cramps and joint pains are not only due to hypothyroidism but are often present due to vitamin D deficiency as well as side-effects from drugs. These drugs include:

Statins (such as Atorvastatin, Simvastatin, Lovastatin, Pravastatin, etc,) which are cholesterol lowering drugs.

<u>Furosemide</u> (brand name Lasix) which is a strong diuretic.
<u>Nifedipine </u>(brand name Procardia) which is used to treat high blood pressure and coronary heart disease.
<u>Donepezil</u> (brand name Aricept) which is used to treat Alzheimer's disease.
<u>Albuterol </u>(brand name Proventil) which is an asthma medicine.
<u>Raloxifene</u> (brand name Evista) which is an anti-osteoporosis drug.

Repeated, strenuous exercise is another common cause of muscle and joint pain.

Dry skin is not only due to hypothyroidism but is also due to dry air caused by air-heating systems during winter months.

Cool skin can be due to poor circulation, in addition to hypothyroidism.

Cold intolerance can be due to the lack of a thick coat of subcutaneous fat in thin, lean individuals.

Puffy eyes are not only due to hypothyroidism, but are often due to sleep deprivation.

Constipation is not only due to hypothyroidism but is often due to less fiber in the diet, old age, depression, diabetes and side-effects from drugs.

Prolonged and excessive menstrual bleeding is often due to uterine fibroids or other disorders affecting the uterus, in addition to hypothyroidism.

Repeated miscarriages can be due to a number of reasons such as stress, older maternal age, autoimmune disorders such as anti-phospholipid syndrome, in addition to Hashimoto's thyroiditis.

A High Prolactin Level can be due to stress, a pituitary tumor, and certain drugs such as Cimetidine, Verapamil, Metoclopramide, etc. Hypothyroidism is only one of the several conditions that can increase prolactin level.

An enlarged thyroid is not always due to Hashimoto's thyroiditis. Graves' disease, thyroid nodules and iodine deficiency are some of the other causes for an enlarged thyroid.

Forgetfullness is not only due to hypothyroidism, but is often present as a result of stress, hardening of the blood vessels of the brain, stroke, diabetes, high blood pressure and vitamin B12 deficiency.

Compression of nerves, such as carpal tunnel syndrome, is not only due to hypothyroidism. Excessive usage of the wrist is a much more common factor.

High blood pressure, cholesterol disorder and leg swelling may not only be due to hypothyroidism. These are common medical conditions in the absence of hypothyroidism.

Slow heart rate may not be due to hypothyroidism. Instead, it may be due to a number of medical conditions, such as a side-effect of a drug or conduction block in the heart, as well as intense cardiovascular aerobic training.

Bottom line: Keep a broader perspective of what may be causing your symptoms.

Chapter **4**

Thyroid Gland and Thyroid Hormones

Now let's take an in-depth look at the structure and function of the thyroid gland. Only then, we will be able to figure out the various causes of hypothyroidism.

What Is The Thyroid?

The Thyroid is an *endocrine* gland. What is an endocrine gland? An endocrine gland is a ductless gland, as compared to a gland with a duct, such as a salivary gland. For instance, a salivary gland delivers its secretion, saliva, through its duct to a local area: in this case, the oral cavity. Glands with ducts are called *exocrine* glands. As compared to an exocrine gland, an endocrine gland secretes its hormone directly into blood circulation, which then exerts its affects on distant organs in the body.

Location

The Thyroid is present in your anterior neck, lying just below the Adam's apple (thyroid cartilage), in front of the trachea (wind-pipe). It moves up with the act of swallowing. If enlarged, you can see it move up with swallowing. That's why your doctor asks you to swallow while inspecting and palpating your thyroid gland.

Structure

The Thyroid gland is shaped like a butterfly. It has two lobes, right and left, with a midline bridge called the isthmus.

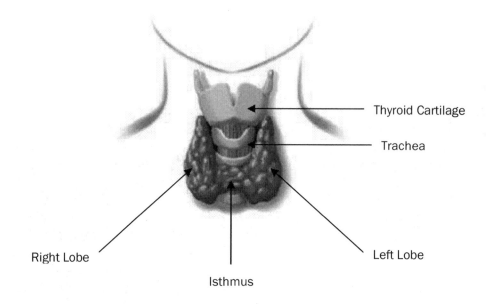

Thyroid Cartilage

Trachea

Right Lobe

Left Lobe

Isthmus

Thyroid

At the microscopic level, the thyroid gland consists of closely packed sacs called follicles. Each follicle is filled with a protein material called colloid. The wall of each follicle is comprised of a single layer of epithelial cells, called follicular cells. These are the cells that produce colloid as well as the thyroid hormones, T4 and T3. T4 is also known as Thyroxine and T3 is also known as Triiodothyronine.

Scattered in between the follicles is another kind of cell called parafollicular cells or C-cells. These cells produce a hormone called Calcitonin, which is involved in the regulation of calcium level in the blood.

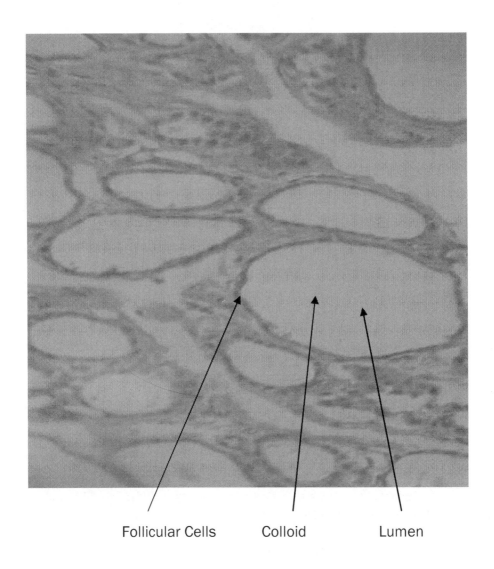

Follicular Cells   Colloid   Lumen

<u>Thyroid Follicles</u>

Function

The primary function of the thyroid gland is to produce two thyroid hormones, T4 and T3. The thyroid follicle is the basic functioning unit of the thyroid gland. Think of a follicle as a sac, lined by a layer of thyroid cells. These are called follicular cells. These cells produce a special protein called Thyroglobulin, which is then stored in the central cavity of each follicle. Synthesis of thyroid hormones takes place on this preformed thyroglobulin.

Synthesis of Thyroid Hormones

Synthesis of thyroid hormones consists of three steps:

1. Iodide Uptake

To synthesize thyroid hormones, thyroid cells need iodine, which primarily comes from diet. Iodine is a trace element which is present in variable amounts in the earth's crust. However, sea water contains fairly good amounts of iodine. Dietary iodine is converted to inorganic iodide inside the body.

Each thyroid cell has an outer (basal) wall, an inner (apical) wall and two sidewalls. The basal wall actively transports iodide from blood circulation into the cell. This is called **Iodide Uptake.** Iodide is then transported inside the thyroid cell towards its inner apical wall, where synthesis of T4 and T3 takes place.

2. Iodination

In order to produce thyroid hormones, the thyroid cell combines iodide with tyrosine, an essential amino acid present inside the thyroglobulin molecule. This process is called **iodination** of tyrosine. This chemical reaction is catalyzed by an enzyme called TPO (Thyroid Peroxidase) as well as H_2O_2 (Hydrogen Peroxide.)

As a result of iodination, two compounds are formed: MIT (Monoiodotyrosine) and DIT (Diiodotyrosine). Each MIT molecule contains one iodide atom and each DIT molecule contains two iodide atoms, attached to tyrosine.

3. Coupling

The next step, called **coupling**, occurs when two DIT molecules fuse to form a molecule that contains four iodide atoms. This is called tetraiodothyronine or thyroxine or T4. Also, one MIT fuses with one DIT, which forms a molecule that contains three iodide atoms. This is called Triiodothyronine or T3. Only T4 and T3 are *true* thyroid hormones. MIT and DIT do not possess any hormonal activity.

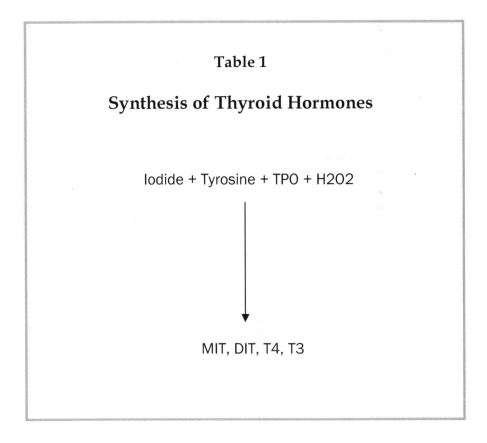

Table 1

Synthesis of Thyroid Hormones

Iodide + Tyrosine + TPO + H2O2

MIT, DIT, T4, T3

Storage

After synthesis, MIT, DIT, T3 and T4 get stored in the thyroglobulin inside the lumen of the follicle. In this way, the thyroid gland serves as a large *reservoir* for storing the thyroid hormones. A normal thyroid gland stores about **8000** microgram of iodine, 90% of which is in the form of MIT, DIT, T3 and T4. The remaining 10% is in the form of iodide.

This unique storage function of the thyroid gland provides a safety-net against depletion of thyroid hormones, should synthesis ceases for some reason.

Release of T4 and T3

Small quantities of T3 and T4 are then released into blood circulation according to your body's needs. This process involves re-absorption of thyroglobulin from the follicular lumen back into the thyroid cell, where thyroglobulin undergoes breakdown. Consequently, T4, T3, DIT and MIT are freed from the thyroglobulin molecule. T3 and T4 are released into blood circulation at the basal wall of the cell. MIT and DIT remain inside the cell and undergo further breakdown, as a result of which *iodide* is freed from tyrosine. A variable amount of freed iodide gets released into blood circulation. The remaining freed iodide stays inside the cell and is recycled for reformation of MIT and DIT.

Under normal circumstances, the thyroid gland releases about **80 - 90** micrograms of T4 and **6 - 8** micrograms of T3 per day.

Transport Of T4 and T3

Most of the T4 and T3 circulate in the blood, tightly bound to proteins, the most important of which is called TBG (Thyroid Binding Globulin). The other two less important binding proteins are TBPA (Thyroid Binding PreAlbumin) and albumin.

T4 and T3 in the bound form are metabolically inactive. Only a tiny fraction, 0.03% of total T4 and 0.3% of total T3, is present as Free T4 and Free T3 respectively. It is these free fractions that are *available* to tissues. Remember, even Free T4 is metabolically *not* very active. It needs to be converted to Free T3, which is the active thyroid hormone.

T4 to T3 Conversion in the Tissues

T3 is the active thyroid hormone, responsible for all of the biological actions of the thyroid hormone. Daily total production of T3 is about **32** micrograms (mcg), about 75-80% (24-26 mcg) of which comes from T4 to T3 conversion in the peripheral tissues. However, about 20-25% (6-8 micrograms) of the total daily production of T3 comes directly from the thyroid gland.

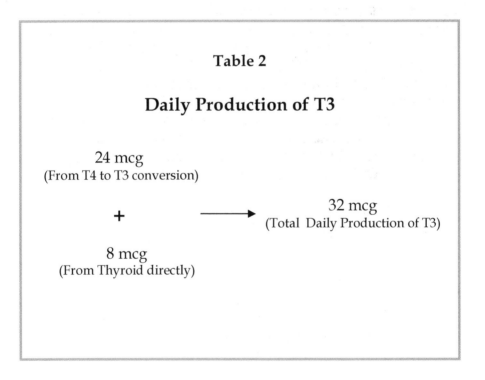

Table 2

Daily Production of T3

24 mcg
(From T4 to T3 conversion)

+ ⟶ 32 mcg
(Total Daily Production of T3)

8 mcg
(From Thyroid directly)

T4 to T3 conversion takes place under the guidance of an enzyme called 5'-deiodinase (DI). There are two types of 5'-DI: Type 1-DI and Type 2-DI. Type 1-DI is most abundant in the peripheral tissues, especially in the thyroid, liver, kidneys and muscles. Type 2-DI is mostly found in the brain and pituitary gland.

T4 Conversion to Inactive Reverse T3

T4 is also converted into an *inactive* form of T3 which is called reverse T3 (rT3). This conversion takes place under the guidance of another enzyme, called 5-deiodinase or Type 3 DI. Daily production of rT3 is about **19** micrograms

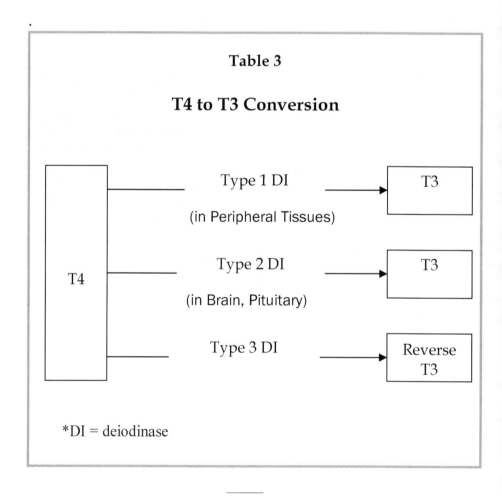

Table 3

T4 to T3 Conversion

T4	Type 1 DI (in Peripheral Tissues) →	T3
	Type 2 DI (in Brain, Pituitary) →	T3
	Type 3 DI →	Reverse T3

*DI = deiodinase

Degradation Of T4 to other Inactive Compounds

About 70% of circulating Free T4 is converted to Free T3 and rT3 in a ratio of about 60% T3 to 40% rT3. The remaining 30% of Free T4 is converted into *Inactive* compounds through mechanisms independent of deiodinases. These mechanisms are sulfation, glucuronidation, deamination and decarboxylation of T4, primarily in the liver. These are called the *alternative* pathways of T4 degradation.

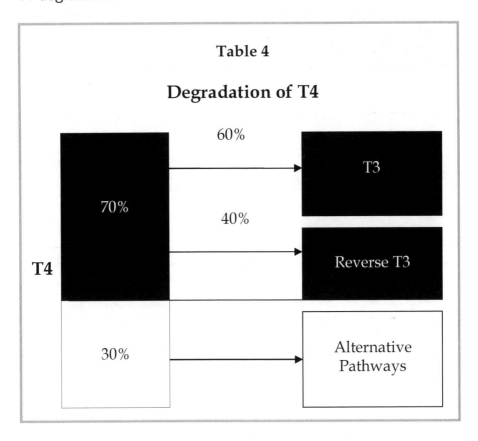

Table 4

Degradation of T4

These *alternative* pathways of T4 degradation become clinically important when someone is on high dose of Levothyroxine. Typically, these are the patients who have undergone total thyroidectomy for thyroid cancer. A high dose of Levothyroxine causes a *shift* to increased T4 *degradation* into inactive compounds through alternative pathways. Consequently, less T4 is left for conversion into T3 (1). Therefore, these individuals suffer from a Low T3 state due to two reasons: a marked *decrease* in the peripheral T4 to T3 conversion and a *lack* of about 20% of daily production of T3 from the thyroid gland itself.

Deiodination means removal of one iodide atom. Each T4 molecule contains 4 atoms of iodide located at 3,3', 5 and 5' positions inside the molecule. Each T3 molecule contains 3 iodide atoms, located at 3, 3', and 5 positions. Each Reverse-T3 molecule contains 3 iodide atoms, located at 3, 3', and 5' positions. T3 and Reverse-T3 are further deiodinated to T2, which is then deiodinated to T1 and ultimately to T0. Clinically speaking, T2, T1 and T0 are believed to contain no significant biologic activity.

T3 is the Active Thyroid Hormone

Out of all of the thyroid hormones, T3 is the *most* active hormone. In order to carry out the thyroid hormone function, T3 combines with Thyroid Hormone Receptor (THR) located inside the nucleus of a cell. T3 exerts its effects on almost every organ in the body, in particular the heart, brain, muscles, bones, skin, intestines and reproductive organs.

Regulation

The function of the thyroid gland is regulated in several ways:

1. The Pituitary Gland regulates thyroid hormone production by producing TSH (Thyroid Stimulating Hormone). The Pituitary Gland senses the level of T3, judges it to be normal, low or high and produces the amount of TSH in an *inverse* manner. In this way, the pituitary produces more TSH if T3 is low, and less TSH if T3 is high.

TSH goes to the thyroid gland and tries to increase or decrease the production of thyroid hormones: high TSH increases and low TSH decreases the production of thyroid hormones.

2. The function of the pituitary gland is regulated by another endocrine gland, called **the hypothalamus,** which is located above the pituitary gland. The hypothalamus regulates the function of the pituitary gland by producing a number of hormones. In terms of thyroid regulation, it produces a hormone called TRH (Thyrotropin Releasing Hormone), which fine-tunes the production of TSH, which in turn regulates the production of thyroid hormones by the thyroid gland.

The hypothalamus itself is influenced by the *limbic* system, as well as various chemicals (neurotransmitters) in the brain. The Limbic system is the center of our emotions. In this way, stress as well as psychiatric illnesses as well as medications can affect the production of your thyroid hormones, by influencing your hypothalamus and pituitary gland.

3. The Thyroid also has an incredible **auto-regulation.** For example, if there is an acute load of a *large* amount of iodine/iodide, the thyroid gland gets *saturated* with the amount of iodine it needs. Subsequently, there is a decrease in the amount of further uptake of iodine/iodide for a few days, after which uptake of iodine resumes normally. A large dose of iodine/iodide also temporarily decreases the release of thyroid hormones into circulation.

These are primarily *protective* mechanisms against the production and release of excessive thyroid hormones in case there is a sudden supply of large quantities of the raw material, iodine/iodide. (For example, contrast agents used during CT scans and angiograms contain huge quantities of iodine). In the same way, cough syrups usually contain large quantities of iodine. Iodine is also used as an antiseptic for skin cuts and wounds. Thanks to the auto-regulatory mechanisms, the vast *majority* of people do not become hyperthyroid or hypothyroid after a large load of iodine.

However, hypothyroidism or hyperthyroidism may *rarely* develop due to the chronic use of iodine in large doses. This has been reported in individuals with pre-existing Hashimoto's thyroiditis or Graves' disease. However, the *vast* majority of people do *not* become *hyperthyroid* or *hypothyroid* if they consume large amounts of iodine. The Japanese are the best evidence in this regard. The average Japanese consumes more than **12,000** micrograms of iodine per day, as compared to the typical American who consumes only about **240** micrograms of iodine per day. The incidence of hyperthyroidism or hypothyroidism is *not* significantly different between these two populations.

Chapter 5

What Is The
Cause Of Your Hypothyroidism?

In order to figure out what is the cause of your hypothyroidism, let's take a look at various causes of hypothyroidism.

Causes of Hypothyroidism in Adults

Stress	Radiation
Obesity	Iodine Deficiency
Aging	Iodine Excess (Rarely)
Any Illness	Selenium Deficiency
Autoimmune Thyroiditis	Goitrogens in Food
Painless Thyroiditis/ Post-Partum Thyroiditis	Thyroid Surgery
Drugs	Pituitary Disorder

Now let's see how various conditions give rise to hypothyroidism. Often, more than one condition is present in a given individual.

How Stress Causes Hypothyroidism

Stress is a major factor that causes hypothyroidism. This is how? Stress causes an increase in serum cortisol, which causes a decrease in Type 1-DI (deiodinase) activity, thereby reducing the T4 to T3 conversion in the tissues. Also, excess serum cortisol has a *negative* effect on TSH production. It prevents the *expected* increase in TSH in response to low T3 level. Therefore, pituitary TSH does *not* get elevated, which prevents an increase in the secretion of T4 and T3 from the thyroid gland, which would occur in the presence of elevated TSH.

Net result: a decrease in T3 in the tissues due to decreased conversion of T4 to T3 which causes hypothyroidism, while TSH and Free T4 remain in the normal range.

You can see how your hypothyroidism due to stress would be easily missed by a physician who simply looks at TSH and Free T4 levels.

Stress is known to cause Hashimoto's thyroiditis. Consequently, synthesis of thyroid hormones go down in the thyroid gland.

****

How Obesity Causes Hypothyroidism

Your thyroid gland produces fairly fixed amounts of thyroid hormones: about 80 - 90 micrograms of T4 and 6-8 micrograms of T3 per day. As you gain weight, you require higher and higher amounts of thyroid hormones, which your thyroid gland cannot supply. Consequently, you start to develop hypothyroidism. As you develop hypothyroidism, your metabolism slows down, which results in weight gain. You get trapped in a *vicious* cycle: Weight gain causing hypothyroidism, and hypothyroidism causing weight gain.

In addition, obesity also causes a decrease in the conversion of T4 to T3. This is how: Obesity is associated with an increase in the production of *cytokines*, which are chemicals produced by the cells of the immune system. These cytokines include Tumor Necrosis Factor- alpha (TNF-alpha), interleukins (IL-1 beta, IL-2 and IL-6), and interferon-gamma (IFN-gamma). Cytokines are known to diminish the activity of Type 1-DI (deiodinase) in peripheral tissues (2). Consequently, there is a decrease in T3 production from T4. A recent provocative study clearly showed that IL-1beta *decreases* the activity of Type 1-DI deiodinase in the liver (3)

In this way, obesity can cause hypothyroidism *via* two mechanisms: a relative decrease in the production of thyroid hormones from the thyroid and a decrease in the production of T3 in the peripheral tissues due to the inhibitory effects of cytokines. You can see how your hypothyroidism due to obesity would be easily missed by a physician who simply looks at TSH and Free T4 levels.

✳✳

How Aging Causes Hypothyroidism

After the age of 60, Type 1-DI (deiodinase) starts to decline, which results in a decrease in T3 formation from T4 in the peripheral tissues. But Free T4 remains normal. Therefore, T4 to T3 conversion in the pituitary gland carried out by Type 2-DI deiodinase remains normal. Consequently, pituitary TSH production also remains normal. Net result: a normal free T4 and TSH (on your blood test), while you are really low in free T3 and experiencing hypothyroidism at the peripheral tissues.

You can see how your hypothyroidism due to old-age would be easily missed by a physician who simply looks at TSH and Free T4 levels.

✳✳

How An Illness Causes Hypothyroidism

Any illness such as infections, uncontrolled diabetes, kidney disease, cirrhosis of liver, surgery, anesthesia, trauma and malnutrition can decrease T4 to T3 conversion in the peripheral tissues. Result: hypothyroidism at the tissue level. In the blood, Free T3 is low and rT3 (reverse T3) is high, while Free T4 and TSH are usually normal.

You can see how your hypothyroidism due to an illness would be easily missed by a physician who simply looks at TSH and Free T4 levels.

****

How Autoimmune Thyroiditis Causes Hypothyroidism

Autoimmune thyroiditis is a condition in which your immune system goes *haywire* and starts to attack your own thyroid gland. If Autoimmune Thyroiditis is associated with an *enlarged* thyroid gland (goiter), it is called **Hashimoto's thyroiditis** (goiterous thyroiditis). On the other hand, if Autoimmune Thyroiditis is present *without* an enlarged thyroid gland, it is called **Atrophic Thyroiditis.**

In Autoimmune Thyroiditis, there is inflammation, destruction and fibrosis (scarring) of the thyroid tissues, which ultimately leads to hypothyroidism.

Genetics and stress are two well-known factors that cause Autoimmune Thyroiditis. I discuss Autoimmune Thyroiditis in more detail in the next chapter.

****

In a lot of individuals, stress, genetics, weight gain and aging work together to cause hypothyroidism. Consider this case scenario:

You have a genetic predisposition to an autoimmune disorder. As an adult, you start to experience more and more stress of daily living. As you age, your metabolism slows down and you start to gain weight, which adds to your stress, especially if you are a female. This ever-increasing stress leads to stress eating behavior and more weight gain. A vicious cycle sets in. Stress also brings out Hashimoto's thyroiditis which you have in your genes. All of these factors act in *concert* and ultimately, make you hypothyroid at the tissue level. Then, you have difficulty losing weight even if you restrict your food intake.

You also usually suffer from tiredness due to hypothyroidism, stress and Vitamin B12 deficiency. If you are a female, you may also have prolonged, heavy menses, which causes iron deficiency and adds to your fatigue. You may also experience thinning of hair and brittle nails.

You mention these symptoms to your physician, who checks your TSH and/or Free T4, which turns out to be normal. Your physician *concludes* that your thyroid is all fine and your symptoms cannot be due to hypothyroidism. At this point, you may also become depressed due to ongoing stress and hypothyroidism, as well as lack of hope from your physician.

****

How Painless Thyroiditis and Postpartum Thyroiditis Causes Hypothyroidism

Painless thyroiditis refers to a condition of *inflammation* of the thyroid gland. However, there is no pain in the thyroid area. Hence, the name Painless Thyroiditis.

Postpartum thyroiditis refers to painless thyroiditis that develops in women after they have delivered a baby.

Symptoms of Painless thyroiditis as well as Postpartum thyroiditis occur in two phases:

Symptoms of hyperthyroidism:

- Restlessness
- Palpitations
- Insomnia/anxiety
- Excessive perspiration
- Intolerance to heat
- Excessive weight loss despite good appetite

A few (6-12) weeks later, these symptoms subside on their own and symptoms of hypothyroidism develop, which typically include:

Symptoms of hypothyroidism:

- Fatigue, sluggishness
- Weight gain
- Intolerance to cold
- Depressed mood

The cause of Painless thyroiditis as well as Postpartum thyroiditis is an inflammation of the thyroid gland, which causes structural damage to the thyroid gland. It's like a tornado hitting a trailer park.

Normally, the thyroid gland stores a large amount of thyroid hormones to be released in small quantities over a period of time.

With the destruction of the gland, the large quantities of the stored thyroid hormones gets released into the blood circulation. This causes the phase of hyperthyroidism.

The thyroid hormones remain in circulation for a few weeks (6-12 weeks) and so does the phase of hyperthyroidism.

After the tornado goes away, the thyroid gland starts to repair itself, but it takes a while. During this period, there is shortage of thyroid hormones, which gives rise to the phase of hypothyroidism. This phase typically last a few weeks (6-12 weeks). Eventually, in most cases, the thyroid gland restores back to normal, although some patients may become hypothyroid permanently.

* *

How Certain Drugs Can Cause Hypothyroidism

Certain drugs can cause hypothyroidism. These drugs include :

Steroids	PTU (PropylThioUracil)
Propranolol	Methimazole

Steroids include
Medrol,
Solu-Medrol
Depo-Medrol (generic methylprednisolone)
Deltasone (generic prednisone)
Decadron (generic dexamethasone)
Cortef (generic hydrocortisone)

Steroids are widely used in clinical practice to treat a number of diseases such as asthma, acute bronchitis, rheumatoid arthritis, allergies, skin rashes, autoimmune disorders and cancer (during chemotherapy).

Steroids interfere with the normal functioning of T1-DI (deiodinase). Consequently, they cause a decrease in the production of T3 in the peripheral tissues and you end up becoming hypothyroid.

In addition, steroids cause a decrease in the production of TSH from the pituitary gland. A decrease in TSH leads to a *decrease* in the production of thyroid hormones by the thyroid gland, which further contributes to the development of hypothyroidism.

On blood testing, your Free T3 is low or low-normal, Free T4 is normal, and your TSH may be low. Consider this: Your physician is trained to order only Free T4 and TSH, and interpret a low TSH as too *much* thyroid hormone. With this mind-set, he/she may decide to decrease the dose of your thyroid hormone. In this way, your physician may actually make you even more hypothyroid, while blindly following the *guidelines* developed by large medical organizations.

Propranolol (Brand name Inderal) is a beta-blocker used for blood pressure control, heart arrhythmias, Migraine headaches and tremors.

Propranolol can interfere with the normal functioning of T1-DI (deiodinase). Consequently, it causes a decrease in the production of T3 in the peripheral tissues and you end up becoming hypothyroid. However, your TSH and Free T4 remain normal. You can see how your hypothyroidism due to Propranolol would be easily missed by a physician who simply looks at TSH and Free T4 levels.

Amiodarone (Brand name Cordarone) is used to treat heart arrhythmias. Amiodarone can also cause hypothyroidism in another way: by causing inflammation and destruction of the thyroid gland.

PTU (PropylThioUracil) is used to treat overactive thyroid in Graves' disease. PTU also decrease synthesis of thyroid hormones in the thyroid gland by inhibiting iodination and coupling.

Methimazole is another drug that is used to treat hyperthyroidism in Graves' disease. It decreases synthesis of thyroid hormone, but does not decrease peripheral T4 to T3 conversion.

Lithium is used to treat bipolar affective disorder. Lithium can inhibit the release of thyroid hormones from the thyroid gland and result in hypothyroidism.

****

How Radiation Causes Hypothyroidism

Radiation in the form of Radioactive Iodine (I-131) can lead to hypothyroidism. Physicians often use Radioactive iodine to treat hyperthyroidism due to Graves' disease. This is a very superficial approach to treat Graves' disease and has a lot of flaws. For in-depth information, read my book, "Graves' Disease and Hyperthyroidism: What You Must Know Before They Zap Your Thyroid With Radioactive Iodine."

Almost everyone who receives radioactive iodine develops permanent hypothyroidism. How? Thyroid cells take up Radioactive iodine in the same way as they normally take up iodide from the blood. But this time, iodide taken up by the thyroid cell is *radioactive* and destroys the cells. It's like thyroid cells *innocently* eat up *poison* called radioactive iodine. Once the thyroid cells are destroyed, hypothyroidism develops.

Radiation fallout after nuclear accidents, such as the Chernobyl nuclear disaster, causes an increase in the incidence of hypothyroidism as well as thyroid cancer in those exposed to radiation. Why? One of the main radioactive material in these nuclear fallouts is radioactive iodine (I-131), which causes destruction of the thyroid gland.

Sometimes, radiation of the neck as a part of a treatment protocol for cancer can give rise to hypothyroidism. Hodgkin's lymphoma is a typical example. However, any radiation exposure of the neck region can increase your risk of hypothyroidism as well as thyroid cancer.

****

How Iodine Deficiency Can Cause Hypothyroidism

Iodine is essential for the normal functioning of the thyroid gland.

As I elaborated earlier, iodine is the raw material for the synthesis of thyroid hormones. Obviously, if you are low in iodine, your thyroid gland has *difficulty* manufacturing normal amounts of thyroid hormones. Low thyroid hormones lead to over-production of TSH (Thyroid Stimulating Hormone) by the pituitary gland. TSH gets in the blood circulation and reaches the thyroid gland, where it stimulates the thyroid gland to produce more thyroid hormones. But your thyroid gland has a hard time doing so, because of deficiency of iodine, the raw material for the synthesis of thyroid hormones. That's how you can develop hypothyroidism due to iodine deficiency.

A high level of TSH also causes your thyroid gland to grow bigger. An enlarged thyroid gland is called a goiter. That's how some individuals with iodine-deficiency eventually end up with goiter and hypothyroidism

How Frequent Is Iodine Deficiency?

World-wide, iodine deficiency is a serious public health crisis. Approximately 40% of the world's population is at risk of iodine deficiency. In certain parts of the world, iodine deficiency is rampant. These areas include the Himalayan slopes, the Andean region of South America, the European Alps and mountainous areas of China and the Rift Valley regions of East and Central Africa.

In countries where salt is iodized, such as the USA, frank iodine deficiency is *presumed* to be rare, although it is now debatable. There is evidence to indicate that iodine deficiency may be more common than endocrinologists have traditionally thought.

An excellent study reported a significant decline in the iodine status of women of child-bearing age in the USA: a surprising 14.9% of women aged 15-44 years and 6.9% of pregnant women had a urinary iodine concentration of 50 micrograms/L, which indicates moderate iodine deficiency (4).

These women had normal levels of TSH and T4 (Thyroxine) in the blood. However, their fetuses were potentially at risk for hypothyroidism, which is quite alarming. It shows how our heavy reliance on TSH and T4 to diagnose hypothyroidism can be misleading.

Iodine requirements increase during pregnancy. For this reason, WHO (World Health Organization) now recommends daily dietary intake of iodine as 250 microgram in pregnant women, as compared to 150 micrograms per day for non-pregnant women (5), in order to avoid hypothyroidism in the newborn.

Some other individuals may be at high risk of iodine deficiency, such as patients on restricted salt intake because of high blood pressure and congestive heart failure. Patients with chronic kidney disease, chronic diarrhea and malnutrition are also at increased risk of iodine deficiency.

In addition, there is an increasing trend towards salt-free and vegan diets for a variety of reasons. Iodine deficiency is quite likely to develop in these individuals. A lot of individuals have replaced iodized salt with sea salt or Himalayan salt, both of which are excellent health choices, as these salts contain about 83 minerals, as compared to iodized salt, which only contains Sodium Chloride and the added Potassium Iodide. However, sea salt contains very little iodine and Himalayan salt contains none. Therefore, if you decide to go on sea salt or Himalayan salt, you need to supplement your iodine from other sources.

How To Diagnose Iodine Deficiency

More than 90% of iodine is excreted through urine. Therefore, you can determine whether or not you have an adequate level of iodine by checking how much iodine you excrete in the urine. The more iodine deficient you are, the more your body will hold onto iodine, which will result in *lesser* amounts of iodine excreted in the urine.

There are various tests to check for iodine deficiency. These include:

- Spot urine test for iodine
- 24-hours urine collection for iodine
- Iodine-Loading Test

In the Spot Urine Test and 24-hour Urine Collection Test, iodine deficiency is defined as follows:

URINARY IODINE CONCENTRATION (microgram/L)	IODINE STATUS
<20	Severe deficiency
20-49	Moderate deficiency
50-99	Mild deficiency

In the **Iodine-Loading Test**, you ingest 50 mg (milligrams) of iodine/iodide, and collect your urine over the next 24-hours for iodine. If you excrete less than 45 mg (90%) of the ingested dose, you are low in iodine (6).

What Are the Natural Sources of Iodine?

Iodine is present in soil and seawater. Animals and plants "eat up" iodine from earth and seawater. Human get iodine by eating these animals and plants. The iodine content of foods varies. In general, seafood has the highest amounts, followed by animal foods. Plants (except seaweeds) have the lowest amounts of iodine.

Good dietary sources of iodine

- Seaweeds
- Fish
- Shrimp

- Iodized salt
- Turkey
- Potatoes with peels
- Milk
- Navy beans

Regular salt does not contain any iodine, but iodized salt is fortified with Potassium iodide, a practice that started in the USA in the 1920's and has effectively reduced the incidence of goiter in this country. One teaspoon of iodized salt contains about **400** micrograms of iodine. Sea salt, on the other hand, has very little iodine, as iodine gets evaporated during the processing of the sea salt. Rock salt and Himalayan salt do not contain any iodine.

How Much Iodine Do You Need?

In the USA, the *recommended* daily amount of iodine is 150 micrograms, although there is a mounting evidence to show that you need more than this recommended dose for your overall health. Recent studies indicate that iodine is not only important for the health of your thyroid gland, but is also vital for the health of other glands, in particular breasts, ovaries, adrenals and prostate.

The daily recommended amount of iodine as 150 micrograms per day was developed to prevent goiter. It appears that you need much more iodine for the optimal health of tissues other than thyroid, such as breasts, ovaries, adrenals and prostate. Currently, this is a new horizon of clinical research. The best clinical evidence is the Japanese population, who have the lowest cancer rates in the world. While there may be several factors why Japanese have low rates of cancer, their diet is rich in iodine, which may be a significant factor for low cancer rate. On an average, a Japanese consumes iodine in the amount of 3,000-12,000 micrograms per day, in the form of seaweeds.

For the general population, a daily iodine intake of 3,000-6,000 micrograms appears to be optimal as well as safe. You can get it in the form of sea-food, seaweeds, iodized salt, iodine supplements, etc.

Why Most Physicians Are Against High Dose Of Iodine

Traditionally, endocrinologists have been taught that if you take iodine and/or iodide in excess of 500 micrograms per day, you could develop hypothyroidism. How? The explanation is thought be due to an *erroneous* concept called the Wolff-Chaikoff effect.

What is the Wolff-Chaikoff effect? In1948, Dr. J Wolff and Dr. I Chaikoff from UC Berkeley published the results of an experiment (7) in healthy rats in which they gave increasing doses of dietary iodine (10-500 microgarms per rat). Then, they gave these rats *radioactive* iodine. Then, they measured the amount of *radioactive* iodine that got incorporated into the thyroid. They found there was a substantial decrease in the amount of *radioactive* iodine found in the thyroid gland, as the dose of *dietary* iodine was increased from 10 to 500 micrograms. They concluded that there was a substantial decrease in the *formation* of thyroid hormone with the increase in the dose of dietary iodine. They extrapolated their findings to conclude that large doses of iodine can cause hypothyroidism and goiter. Later, Dr. Wolff extrapolated these findings to humans in an editorial in the prestigious *American Journal of Medicine* (8). At that time, he was a famous physician at NIH (National Institute of Health.) Since then, the Wolff-Chaikoff effect became an absolute basic law in medicine. Every physician learns and abides by it. That's why physicians in general, are reluctant to use high doses of dietary iodine.

However, I find the Wolff-Chaikoff effect to be an outdated, erroneous concept. Here is my explanation. Dr. Wolff and Chaikoff *mistakenly* presumed the rats got hypothyroid because rats had less radioiodine uptake by their thyroid gland. But this is *not* how we diagnose hypothyroidism.

To diagnose someone with hypothyroidism, you need a blood test, not a radioiodine scan. Dr. Wolff and Chaikoff did *not* do a blood test for thyroid function in their rats, because these blood tests were probably not available at that time. The low radioiodine uptake happened because a large dose of dietary iodine *saturated* the thyroid gland. That's why thyroid glands of these rats took up only a small amount of subsequently administered radio-iodine. This is a perfectly normal response. It does not indicate that the rats became hypothyroid.

In fact, there are a number of situations where radioiodine uptake of thyroid is low, but these individuals are NOT hypothyroid. For example, if you have a CT scan of a part of your body done for some reason and a few days later, if you have a radioiodine scan of your thyroid, it will show low radioiodine uptake. But your blood test for thyroid would be unaffected. For this reason, you should wait at least 2-4 weeks after any diagnostic procedure that uses a contrast agent to have a thyroid scan Why? Because contrast agents have a high amount of iodine, which *saturates* the iodine pool of your body for several weeks, including your thyroid gland, which closes its door for any more iodine to come in. Therefore, if you have a radioiodine uptake of the thyroid, it will be low, but your blood test for thyroid will be normal. Hence, you will not be hypothyroid. By the mishap of luck, if you lived in the 1950's and happened to be a patient of Dr. Wolff or Dr. Chaikoff, you would *erroneously* be diagnosed as having hypothyroidism.

I am not alone in my conclusions that the Wolf-Chaikoff concept is erroneous. Several other out-of-the-box physicians have reached the same conclusion. One such noteworthy physician is Dr. G.E. Abraham, a retired professor of Obstetrics, Gynecology, and Endocrinology at UCLA. In a thought-provoking article (9), he critically analyzes the Wolff-Chaikoff effect and reaches the same conclusion that the legendary Wolff-Chaikoff effect is indeed an erroneous concept.

In fact, iodine in high doses was a standard medical practice in the later half of the 19th century and the first half of the 20th century. High dose iodine was used to treat a number of medical conditions, notably goiter, bronchitis, Scarlet fever , Tuberculosis, etc. Then, iodine-use went out of favor due to the highly publicized Wolff-Chaikoff effect.

In the last decade, there has been a resurgence in the use of iodine in high doses. Thousands of people consume iodine/iodide in large amounts, as iodine has been shown to be an important nutrient for the health of every cell, in particular thyroid, breast, ovaries, adrenals, brain and skin. Grass-root discussion groups have formed on the internet, in which patients share their stories about the healing effects of iodine.

It is interesting to note that the Japanese have traditionally used high amounts of iodine in the form of seaweeds. On an average , a Japanese person roughly consumes anywhere from 3000 mcg to 12,000 mcg of iodine per day. Compare this to RDA (Recommended Daily Allowance) in the US which is 150 mcg. The Japanese do not have a higher incidence of hypothyroidism as compared to other populations. Interestingly, they do have a much *lower* incidence of breast and prostate cancer, cardiovascular mortality and infant deaths as compared to the US population. Could it be due to high iodine consumption?

****

Can High-Dose Iodine Cause Thyroid Problems?

There are only *rare* reports in medical literature incriminating high-dose iodine to hypothyroidism or hyperthyroidism. These rare cases happen in individuals with autoimmune thyroid disease such as Hashimoto's thyroiditis or Graves' disease or those who have a nodular goiter.

In 2011, one such case was reported: an 82-year-old Japanese man developed severe hypothyroidism triggered by absorption of iodine from an iodine-containing skin ointment used in diabetic gangrene treatment (10).

A common case *scenario* goes like this: You are on a thyroid hormone pill for your hypothyroidism and see your regular physician every 6-12 months. In the meantime, you also see your *naturopath*, who places you on high doses of iodine supplement. Your regular physician may not order your thyroid function test for several months. During this time, you may become hyperthyroid (or rarely hypothyroid).

Therefore, if you decide to consume large amounts of iodine, let your regular health care professional know about it. More importantly, make sure you have a blood test for Free T3, Free T4 and TSH every 2-3 months.

****

How Selenium Deficiency Can Cause Hypothyroidism

Selenium is a mineral that we need in small quantities to stay healthy. Selenium is especially important for the normal functioning of the thyroid gland. In fact, selenium is most abundant in the thyroid as compared to any other organ in the body. Selenium is also important for the normal functioning of Type 1 deiodinase, the enzyme that is responsible for the conversion of T4 to T3 in the peripheral tissues.

Selenium deficiency, therefore can lead to a decrease in T3 level and consequently, causes hypothyroidism. Selenium deficiency can also cause goiter formation, especially if you are also low in iodine.

In addition to thyroid health, selenium is also important for the health of the immune system, cardiovascular system, reproductive system and the brain. It also seems to reduce the risk of cancer, especially prostate cancer.

Who is at Risk of Selenium Deficiency?

Selenium deficiency is **uncommon** in the general population. However, some individuals are at high risk of selenium deficiency due to life-style and medical conditions, which includes:

- Vegetarianism/Veganism
- Gluten-free diets
- Malabsorption due to Crohn's disease, Ulcerative Colitis, Celiac disease, intestinal resection/bypass surgery.
- HIV
- Kidney dialysis
- Statins (Cholesterol lowering drugs) in some individuals

Selenium and iodine deficiencies have interesting relationships: Severe hypothyroidism and cretinism (childhood mental retardation) develops in individuals low in both iodine and selenium. If you start to supplement iodine, selenium deficiency worsens. Conversely, iodine deficiency worsens if you start to supplement with selenium alone. Therefore, both, iodine as well as selenium, should be supplemented concurrently.

Selenium deficiency can be diagnosed on a blood test.

How much Selenium Do You Need?

The Recommended Daily Allowance (RDA) of selenium for adults is 55 mcg (micrograms).

The upper safe limit is considered to be 400 mcg per day. However, some studies have used doses up to 600 mcg per day without any side-effects. Most studies have used daily doses of 100-300 mcg. Many experts in the field recommend a daily dose of 200 mcg.

Natural Sources Of Selenium

Selenium in found in soil, but its amount varies. Consequently, its amount in plants and animals also varies from place to place. Various parts of China are the world's most selenium-deficient regions in the world. In the USA, the Northeast and Northwest have low selenium as compared to the Midwest and Southwest.

Brazil nuts are the single best natural source of selenium, followed by organ meats (Liver, kidneys), Tuna, Halibut, Sardines, shellfish, beef, turkey and chicken. A Brazil nut can provide you with an amazing amount of 70-90 mcg of selenium.
Selenium is also present in *decent* amounts in whole grains, eggs and cereals.

Selenium Toxicity

Too much of anything causes toxicity and so does selenium excess. Early signs of selenium toxicity include a garlic odor and a metallic taste. The clinical features of chronic selenium toxicity include diarrhea, nausea, hair loss, brittle nails, mottled teeth, and neurological symptoms.

****

How Certain Foods Can Cause Hypothyroidism

Some plant-foods contain chemicals that can interfere with the synthesis of the thyroid hormones. These chemicals are called **goitrogens**, as these chemicals can lead to the formation of a goiter.

Goitrogens interfere with the synthesis of thyroid hormones either by decreasing the uptake of Iodide or by interfering with the process of iodination and coupling.

Foods that contain goitrogens include:
- Cabbages
- Turnips
- Rutabaga
- Kale
- Maize (corn)
- Soy
- Sweet potatoes
- Bamboo shoots
- Cassava meal

Food goitrogens can cause goiter formation and possibly hypothyroidism if you consume goitrogenic foods in *large* amounts and if you have iodine-deficiency.

* *

How Thyroid Surgery Can Cause Hypothyroidism

Thyroid surgery comes in two forms:

- Removal of one side of the thyroid gland
- Removal of the total (or near total) thyroid gland

After total thyroid resection, you develop hypothyroidism as there is no more thyroid hormone production in your body. You have to be on thyroid hormone pills for the rest of your life, without which you will not be able to survive.

Physicians are *diligent* in prescribing thyroid hormone pills to anyone who undergoes total thyroid gland resection. However, this is *not* the case if you have only one half of the thyroid gland removed. Often, physicians do not prescribe thyroid hormone pills for this type of patient. Why? Because there is an *erroneous* concept that one half of the thyroid gland is enough to take care of your thyroid hormone needs. In fact, it is not true.

In reality, what happens is that the remaining half of the thyroid gland enlarges, desperately trying to increase the production of thyroid hormone. But even then, the production of thyroid hormone remains suboptimal. Consequently, you suffer from hypothyroidism.

In addition, the remaining, enlarged half of the thyroid gland often ends up having thyroid nodules, which is the reason you had your other half of the thyroid removed in the first place. Then, you restart the cycle of repeated thyroid ultrasounds and biopsies, all of which can be avoided if your physician places you on thyroid hormone soon after thyroid surgery.

Therefore, I place my patients on thyroid hormone pills after they undergo any extent of thyroid surgery: partial or total.

****

Secondary Hypothyroidism/Tertiary Hypothyroidism

Hypothyroidism can result due to disorders of the pituitary, which causes a decrease in the production of TSH. Low TSH leads to low production of thyroid hormones by the thyroid gland. That's why it is called **secondary hypothyroidism** as compared to *primary* hypothyroidism, which is due to disorders of the thyroid gland.

A disorder of the hypothalamus can lead to a low TSH production by the pituitary and subsequent hypothyroidism. This is called **tertiary hypothyroidism.**

The most common cause of secondary/tertiary hypothyroidism is the use of steroids. As I explained earlier, steroids have an *inhibitory* effect on the production of TSH. Consequently, the TSH level goes down, which results in secondary/tertiary hypothyroidism.

Steroids include:
Medrol,
Solu-Medrol
Depo-Medrol (generic methylprednisolone)
Deltasone (generic prednisone)
Decadron (generic dexamethasone)
Cortef (generic hydrocortisone)

These drugs are widely used in clinical practice to treat a number of diseases such as asthma, acute bronchitis, rheumatoid arthritis, allergies, skin rashes, autoimmune disorders and cancer (during chemotherapy).

Other medical conditions that give rise to *secondary* hypothyroidism include a large pituitary tumor, infections or acute hemorrhagic necrosis of the pituitary gland. More commonly, the function of the pituitary gland goes down in people who undergo surgery or radiation to the pituitary area, usually to treat tumors in this area of the brain. In these individuals, not only TSH, but other hormones of the pituitary gland also go down, which results in adrenal insufficiency, growth hormone deficiency, low testosterone and low sperm count in men, and inability to lactate, lack of menses and infertility in women.

References:

1. Refetoff S, Nicoloff J, Thyroid hormone transport and metabolism. Endocrinology/edited by Leslie DeGroot et al, Vol.1, 3rd edition. W.B. Saunders Company, 1995.

2. Jakobs TC, Mentrup B, Schmutzler C, Dreher I, Köhrle J. Proinflammatory cytokines inhibit the expression and function of human type I 5'-deiodinase in HepG2 hepatocarcinoma cells. *Eur J Endocrinol*. 2002 Apr;146(4):559-66.

3. Koenig RJ. Regulation of type 1 iodothyronine deiodinase in health and disease. *Thyroid*. 2005 Aug;15(8):835-40.

4. Hollowell JG, Haddow JE. The prevalence of iodine deficiency in women of reproductive age in the United States of America. *Public Health Nutr*. 2007 Dec;10(12A):1532-9

5. Zimmermann MB. Iodine deficiency in pregnancy and the effects of maternal iodine supplementation on the offspring: a review. *Am J Clin Nutr*. 2009 Feb;89(2):668S-72S

6. The Iodine/Iodide Loading Test.
http://www.optimox.com/pics/Iodine/loadTest.htm#2

7. Wolff J, Chaikoff IL.The inhibitory action of excessive iodide upon the synthesis of diiodotyrosine and of thyroxine in the thyroid gland of the normal rat. *Endocrinology.* 1948 Sep;43(3):174-9.

8. Wolff J. Iodide goiter and the pharmacologic effects of excess iodide. *Am J Med.* 1969 Jul;47(1):101-24.

9. Abraham, G.E. The Wolff-Chaikoff Effect: Crying Wolf?
http://www.optimox.com/pics/Iodine/IOD-04/IOD_04.html#1

10. Hayashi M, Onodera K, Suzuki K, Kataoka Y, Tachikawa K, Riku S, Tanaka H. A case of consciousness disturbance resulting from severe hypothyroidism due to chronic thyroiditis and excess iodine absorption. *Intern Med.* 2011;50(21):2627-32.

Chapter **6**

What is Hashimoto's Thyroiditis, Chronic Autoimmune Thyroiditis and How Do You Diagnose It?

Hashimoto's thyroiditis is an autoimmune disease of the thyroid gland. However, not every case of autoimmune disease of the thyroid is due to Hashimoto's thyroiditis.

Autoimmune disease of the thyroid gland can manifest with hypothyroidism (underactive thyroid), hyperthyroidism (overactive thyroid) or euthyroidism (normal thyroid function).

When an autoimmune disease causes hypothyroidism, it is due to a process called chronic autoimmune thyroiditis. In chronic autoimmune thyroiditis, there is inflammation, destruction and fibrosis (scarring) of the thyroid tissues.

If chronic autoimmune thyroiditis is associated with an *enlarged* thyroid gland (goiter), it is called Hashimoto's thyroiditis (goiterous thyroiditis). On the other hand, if chronic autoimmune thyroiditis is present *without* an enlarged thyroid gland, it is called chronic atrophic thyroiditis.

Not every case of chronic autoimmune thyroiditis (both Hashimoto's as well as atrophic) is associated with hypothyroidism. Some patients go through an initial period of euthyroidism, when their thyroid function is normal. However, ultimately almost all cases of chronic autoimmune thyroiditis end up with hypothyroidism, unless you take active action, which I describe later in the book.

Rarely, a patient with chronic autoimmune thyroiditis can develop hyperthyroidism, called Hashi-toxicosis.

Diagnosis of Chronic Autoimmune Thyroiditis

Chronic autoimmune thyroiditis affects women much more frequently than men at a ratio of about 6:1.

A family history of thyroid disorder or some other autoimmune disorder such as Type 1 diabetes, Asthma, Vitiligo, Rheumatoid arthritis, Celiac disease, Chronic autoimmune gastritis, Myasthenia gravis, Lupus, etc. is usually present. Often, more than one autoimmune disorder is present in the same person.

An enlarged thyroid gland, known as a goiter, is present in about 40-50% of cases. Sometimes, thyroid nodules are present.

Diagnosis of chronic autoimmune thyroiditis can easily be made by a blood test: TPO (Thyroid Peroxidase) antibodies and TG (Thyroglobulin) antibodies are elevated in about 90% of patients with chronic autoimmune thyroiditis.

Non-Destructive Autoimmune Thyroid Disease

Sometimes, autoimmune thyroid disease does not cause tissue destruction of the thyroid. Instead, hypothyroidism is due to an antibody that prevents TSH from acting on its receptors on the thyroid cells. This antibody is called Thyrotropin Receptor Stimulation Blocking Antibody.

To diagnose this condition, you need a special test called TBII (Thyrotropin Binding Inhibit Immunoglobulin).

You can get rid of these antibodies and cure your hypothyroidism by adhering to my treatment strategy for immune dysfunction, discussed later in this book.

Other Forms of Chronic Autoimmune Thyroiditis

There are three other forms of chronic autoimmune thyroiditis

- Painless Thyroiditis
- Post-partum Thyroiditis
- Drug-induced thyroiditis

Painless Thyroiditis/Silent Thyroiditis

Painless thyroiditis refers to a condition of inflammation of the thyroid gland. It is called painless thyroiditis to distinguish it from another inflammatory condition of the thyroid called subacute thyroiditis, which causes a lot of pain in the neck. Painless Thyroiditis is also called Silent Thyroiditis.

Painless thyroiditis has a clinical course of several months. Usually, it is triggered by stress and an acute upper respiratory tract infection (URI), such as a common cold.

Symptoms Occur in Two Phases:

Symptoms of hyperthyroidism are followed by symptoms of hypothyroidism.

Symptoms of hyperthyroidism include:

- Restlessness
- Palpitations
- Insomnia/anxiety
- Excessive perspiration
- Intolerance to heat
- Excessive weight loss despite good appetite

A few (6-12) weeks later, these symptoms subside on their own and symptoms of hypothyroidism develop, which typically include:

- Fatigue, sluggishness
- Weight gain
- Intolerance to cold
- Depressed mood

What Causes Painless Thyroiditis?

The cause of Painless thyroiditis is an inflammation of the thyroid gland, which causes *structural* damage to the thyroid gland. It's like a tornado hitting a trailer park.

Normally, the thyroid gland stores a large amount of thyroid hormones to be released in small quantities over a period of time.

With the destruction of the gland caused by the *tornado* of Painless thyroiditis, the large quantities of the stored thyroid hormones gets released into blood circulation. This causes the phase of hyperthyroidism.

The thyroid hormones remain in circulation for a few weeks (6-12 weeks) and so does the phase of hyperthyroidism.

After the tornado goes away, the thyroid gland starts to repair itself, but it takes awhile. During this period, there is a *shortage* of thyroid hormones, which gives rise to the phase of hypothyroidism. This phase typically last a few weeks (6-12 weeks).

Eventually, in most cases, the thyroid gland restores back to normal, although some patients may become hypothyroid permanently if underlying autoimmune dysfunction is not treated. I discuss how to treat autoimmune dysfunction later in the book.

Diagnosis of Painless Thyroiditis

Diagnosis of Painless thyroiditis is a tricky one. Patients usually consult their family physicians, who often do not think about the possibility of Painless thyroiditis.

Patients get placed on a variety of medicines to control their symptoms. Patients do not get better and feel quite frustrated. Usually, it takes an endocrinologist to diagnose Painless thyroiditis.

Diagnostic Tests include:

- Free T4, Free T3 and TSH
- Thyroid Antibodies tests
- Thyroid Radioiodine uptake and scan

Thyroid Radioiodine uptake and scan is the most useful tool in deciding whether hyperthyroidism is due to Painless thyroiditis or Graves' disease. In Painless thyroiditis, radioiodine uptake is minimal. On the other hand, it is elevated in Graves' disease.

The Thyroid Radioiodine uptake and scan should *not* be done if a patient is pregnant or breast-feeding.

Treatment of Painless Thyroiditis

Symptoms of hyperthyroidism can be managed with a Beta-Blocker such as atenolol or propranolol.

Symptoms of hypothyroidism may require a short course of thyroid hormone replacement with T4 and T3.

Patients often continue to have recurrences of bouts of hyperthyroidism followed by hypothyroidism, unless they follow the specific treatment of autoimmune thyroiditis, as discussed later in the book.

Postpartum Thyroiditis

Postpartum thyroiditis refers to thyroiditis that develops in a woman a few weeks after she has delivered a baby.

Its clinical course, diagnosis and treatment is similar to that of Painless thyroiditis.

Diagnosis of postpartum thyroiditis is a tricky one. Patients usually consult their obstetrician or family physician who often do not think about the possibility of postpartum thyroiditis. They blame symptoms of hyperthyroidism on anxiety of motherhood and symptoms of hypothyroidism on postpartum depression.

Patients get placed on a variety of medicines to control their symptoms. Patients do not get better and feel quite frustrated.

Caution:

The radio-iodine uptake and scan should NOT be done if a patient is breast-feeding because of the risk of transmitting radiation to the baby through milk. In that case, clinical monitoring is usually the best option, as hyperthyroidism due to postpartum thyroiditis usually resolves in 6-12 weeks, but does not resolve in the case of Graves' disease.

If it is important to get a diagnosis on an urgent basis, then either the mother can decide to stop breast feeding or pump and store about 5-7 days supply of her breast milk in a refrigerator. By that time, it is safe to resume breast feeding.

Drug-Induced Thyroiditis

Occasionally, drugs can give rise to autoimmune thyroiditis. Amiodarone and interferon are the most *notorious* drugs in this regard, although this list keeps getting longer with the use of newer drugs which act by modifying the immune system.

The clinical course, diagnosis and treatment of Drug Induced Thyroiditis is similar to that of Painless thyroiditis

"Burnt Out" Thyroid In Patients With Graves' Disease

Autoimmune thyroid disease can produce antibodies that stimulate the thyroid cells to produce too much thyroid hormone, or hyperthyroidism, called Graves' disease. These antibodies are called Thyroid Stimulating Immunoglobulins (or TSI).

In patients with Graves' disease, if autoimmune dysfunction is not treated, as almost always is the case, then these patients can develop chronic autoimmune thyroiditis, a destructive process that can eventually destroy most of the thyroid gland. Clinically, we refer to it as the burnt out thyroid gland, which then leads to hypothyroidism in these patients.

Chapter **7**

Diagnosis of Hypothyroidism

The diagnosis of hypothyroidism is often delayed. As I explained earlier, hypothyroidism develops insidiously. Often, patients get used to their symptoms such as fatigue, cold intolerance and inability to lose weight. The exception to this general rule is the patient who undergoes surgical removal of the entire thyroid gland. In such patients, symptoms of hypothyroidism develop rapidly, usually within 3 weeks.

Another common reason why the diagnosis of hypothyroidism is delayed is the heavy reliance on TSH (Thyroid Stimulating Hormone), a laboratory blood test, by physicians to diagnose hypothyroidism. As I explained earlier, TSH tells you what is going on at the level of the pituitary and *not* necessarily what is going on in the peripheral tissues such as muscles, skin, bones, intestines, heart and liver. Therefore, you may have muscle aches and pains, weight gain, fatigue, thinning of hair and many other symptoms of hypothyroidism, but your TSH may still be normal due to a variety of reasons discussed earlier. If your TSH is not elevated, your physician will *discard* the possibility of hypothyroidism as the cause of your symptoms.

Even when your TSH *finally* gets elevated, if your T4 is in the normal range, your physician will likely diagnose you with Subclinical Hypothyroidism, even though you may suffer from fatigue, weight gain, muscles aches and pains and many other symptoms of hypothyroidism. Sad, but true! Physicians generally do not treat Subclinical Hypothyroidism. In the end, you as a patient continue to suffer from hypothyroidism.

In order to diagnose hypothyroidism accurately, your physician needs to carefully *listen* to your symptoms. Obviously, it takes time, a knowledgeable mind and a skillful ear. As I explained earlier, hypothyroidism can affect every single organ in your body. Please refer to Chapter 2, "What are the Symptoms of Hypothyroidism?"

Next, your physician should carry out a thorough physical examination, paying particular attention to the signs of hypothyroidism, which include:

- General appearance may show lethargy, apathy, or slow thinking.
- Weight gain
- Elevated diastolic blood pressure
- Slow pulse
- Temperature may be slightly subnormal
- Thinning of hair, especially at the lateral 1/3rd of the eyebrows.
- Coarse facial features
- Peri-orbital (around eyes) puffiness
- Thick tongue
- Goiter (enlarged thyroid gland)
- Hoarseness of voice
- Heart sounds may be muffled and distant due to "flabby heart muscle" and/or pericardial effusion (fluid around heart)
- Cold hands and feet
- Puffiness of the dorsum of hands and feet
- Lower Leg edema, which is a non-pitting type. It does *not* indent after pressure with a finger.
- Tendon reflexes, (such as knee jerk reflex) have a *slow* relaxation phase. Hence the term, "hung-up" reflexes.

Diagnostic Testing

All you need is a blood test for Free T3 (Free Triiodothyronine), Free T4 (Free Thyroxine), TSH (Thyroid Stimulating Hormone), TG (Thyroglobulin) antibodies and TPO (Thyroid Peroxidase) antibodies. Sometimes, a thyroid ultrasound may be needed if your physician discovers nodule/nodules in your thyroid gland.

In a typical case of *advanced* hypothyroidism, Free T4 and Free T3 are low and TSH is high. As you recall, Free T3 and Free T4 come from the thyroid gland. In addition, T4 gets converted into T3 in the peripheral tissues as well as inside the pituitary gland. Your pituitary gland senses the level of T3, and assesses it to be normal, low or high. Then, it responds by producing TSH in a reciprocal manner: High TSH production if T3 is low, and *vice versa,* low TSH if T3 is high.

In many cases of *early or mild* hypothyroidism, Free T3 is low or low normal, Free T4 is normal and TSH is normal or slightly elevated.

As opposed to TSH, Free T3 truly reflects what is going on inside the peripheral tissues. This is your true *active* thyroid hormone. Free T4 is the *precursor* for Free T3. *Therefore, Free T3 is the single best test to diagnose hypothyroidism.* For optimal thyroid hormone functioning, Free T3 should be more than 3.0 pg/ml in most individuals.

Many individuals have clinical features of hypothyroidism while their Free T4 is in the normal range, TSH is between 2-4 mIU/L and Free T3 is in the low normal range. In these patients, I find their symptoms of hypothyroidism disappear once they receive appropriate treatment.

TG antibodies and/or TPO antibodies are elevated in patients with Hashimoto's Thyroiditis, which is a common cause of hypothyroidism. Rarely, a patient has hypothyroidism and Hashimoto's Thyroiditis clinically, but TG and TPO antibodies are negative. In these cases, the physician should order a blood test for TBII (Thyrotropin Binding Inhibit Immunoglobulin), which, if elevated, indicates an autoimmune thyroid disease, as I discussed earlier in Chapter 6 on Hashimoto's Thyroiditis.

In *secondary/tertiary* hypothyroidism due to pituitary/hypothalamic causes, Free T3 and Free T4 are low or low normal range, and TSH is *not* elevated. It is usually in the normal range or may even be low.

A thyroid ultrasound is a good way to evaluate a thyroid nodule in more detail. If a nodule is more than 1 cm, most thyroidologists in the USA would recommend an ultrasound-guided FNA (Fine Needle Aspiration) biopsy to rule out any malignancy.

Section 2

Treating
and
Curing Hypothyroidism

Chapter **8**

Why The Usual Approach To Treat Hypothyroidism Is Suboptimal

The usual treatment approach for hypothyroidism recommends treating every hypothyroid patient with one approach: Give T4 (Levothyroxine, brand names Synthroid, Levoxyl, Unithroid, Levothroid). We can call it the T4-only hypothesis.

There are a lot of problems with this T4-only hypothesis. Often, it does not truly take care of symptoms, because the approach itself is suboptimal and unscientific. Why?

1. There are various causes of hypothyroidism. Therefore, one-size-fits-all is obviously an unscientific approach. Like other medical conditions, every person with hypothyroidism needs a individualized and *not* a monolithic, computerized approach.

2. T4-alone hypothesis aims to replenish low T4-state, while hypothyroidism is caused by low T3-state. The scientific fact: T4, even Free T4, does not carry out thyroid function inside the cell. It is simply a substrate for the formation of T3 in the tissues. Then, T3 binds to the Thyroid Hormone Receptor (THR), located inside the nucleus of the cells, and carries out the thyroid hormone action. In the nucleus, all you see is T3 and *no* T4. That's why T3 and *not* T4 is the true Active Thyroid hormone.

3. T4-alone hypothesis makes a big presumption that T4 to T3 conversion proceeds normally in the peripheral tissues, in every individual, without even checking if it really is the case. Very unscientific, isn't it?!

4. The scientific fact is that T4 to T3 conversion in the peripheral tissues depends on the normal functioning of an enzyme called Type 1 Deiodinase, which often does *not* function normally due to a variety of common conditions, such as stress, obesity, aging, diabetes, nutritional issues and certain medications including beta-blockers and steroids.

5. In normal individuals, about 20% of the daily production of T3 comes from the Thyroid gland itself and about 80% from the peripheral conversion of T4 to T3. Obviously, the T4-only hypothesis does not take into account this very basic scientific fact.

6. T4-alone hypothesis recommends simply following serum TSH as the gold standard for the adequacy of thyroid hormone replacement, which can be an *incorrect* and *misleading* approach in a lot of individuals. Why? The scientific fact is that TSH production in the pituitary gland depends upon normal functioning of the pituitary gland as well as normal functioning of an enzyme called Type 2 Deiodinase, which is responsible for the T4 to T3 conversion inside the pituitary gland. It is this T3 production inside the pituitary that is the main regulator of TSH production. In a lot of hypothyroid individuals, peripheral conversion of T4 to T3 is *low* due to sub-optimally functioning Type 1 Deiodinase. But their Type 2 Deiodinase functions normally, producing adequate amounts of T3 from T4 inside the Pituitary. Subsequently, TSH production is normal in these individuals, while their peripheral tissues are hypothyroid. *In other words, your pituitary is normal, but your peripheral tissues are actually hypothyroid.* In this way, the current T4-only therapy treats the pituitary test (TSH) and not the patient and their hypothyroidism in the peripheral tissues.

7. Sometimes, even the Pituitary gland is not working normally for a variety of reasons, and does not produce adequate amounts of TSH even when a patient is clearly hypothyroid. This can utterly confuse most physicians who have the mind-set that a low TSH *always* means too much thyroid hormone. Consequently, the physician may even decrease the dose of the patients' thyroid hormone, thus making the poor patient even more hypothyroid.

8. Normally, a low Free T4 due to primary hypothyroidism leads to decreased production of intra-thyroidal T3, which causes an increase in TSH production, which, in turn, causes an increase secretion of T3 from the thyroid gland. However, when such a person is given T4-only therapy to normalize their TSH, their TSH-stimulated increase in T3 secretion goes away. Net effect is a decrease in total circulating T3 level and ongoing hypothyroidism. So the patient actually feels worse after they get placed on T4-only therapy, although their physician is satisfied because their TSH is now normal. I have heard so many hypothyroid patients say that their "life has gone downhill" ever since they were placed on Levothyroxine (Synthroid, Levoxyl).

9. In order to treat a patient's symptoms, physicians usually keep increasing the dose of Levothyroxine (T-4) to the point that the serum T4 level gets close to the upper limit. However, the patient continues to suffer from symptoms of hypothyroidism, which may even get worse. Obviously, this frustrates both the patient and the physician.

Why do your symptoms of hypothyroidism fail to improve or even get worse when you are on a *high* dose of T4-only treatment? Because Type 2 Deiodinase not only converts T4 to T3 inside your pituitary, but is also responsible for T4 to T3 conversion in the brain and the hypothalamus. Now consider this. Your *appetite* center is located inside the hypothalamus. Due to a high level of T3 inside your hypothalamus, your appetite may get into *turbo* charge, causing you to gain more weight. In addition, a high level of T3 inside your brain can lead to anxiety and insomnia, which leads to day-time fatigue and somnolence.

10. The current treatment approach is superficial, even in the hands of those cutting-edge health care professionals who treat hypothyroidism with a combination of T4 and T3. Why? Because even this approach simply aims to treat low thyroid hormone, without treating the underlying root cause of hypothyroidism. As I explained earlier, obesity, stress and autoimmune dysfunction are three major causes of hypothyroidism. These underlying factors often remain untreated, even if a patient is on a T4 and T3 combination therapy. Therefore, the patient continues to suffer and doesn't feel well.

Chapter **9**

My Scientific Approach to Treat and Cure Hypothyroidism

My scientific approach to treat and cure hypothyroidism consists of three steps:

1. Treat Hypothyroidism with T4 and T3
2. Keep a broader perspective
3. Treat the Underlying Cause

Treat Hypothyroidism with T4 and T3

A person develops hypothyroidism due to low T3 in the peripheral tissues, such as skin, muscles, intestines, bones, heart, etc. T3 comes from two sources: directly from the thyroid gland as well as from T4 in the peripheral tissues where T4 converts into T3. In many patients, this T4 to T3 conversion is *not* optimal.

Obviously, a hypothyroid patient needs T4 as well as T3 to replace their deficiency of thyroid hormones. It is so scientific, isn't it? I have been using this approach to treat my hypothyroid patients since 1999, with some amazing results. All of my patients feel better once they are on a combination of T4 and T3. In many, their long-standing symptoms of hypothyroidism finally disappear. Often they ask, " Why don't other doctors use this approach? It makes so much sense and it works." That's one reason why I decided to write this book: to share my clinical experience with other physicians.

Various Preparations of T4 and T3

1. Armour Thyroid or Nature-Throid or Westhroid-P or NP Thyroid

These are various names of the same basic preparation: *desiccated thyroid gland*, usually from pork, or from pork and beef. The thyroid glands are dried (desiccated), ground to powder, combined with binder chemicals known as fillers, and pressed into pills. These are pretty *inexpensive* pills and work very well.

These preparations have been around since the late 19th century and were the standard treatment for hypothyroidism until the 1960's when synthetic T4 hit the market as Synthroid. Gradually, synthetic T4 took over and Synthroid became synonymous with "hypothyroidism treatment" due to effective marketing by the pharmaceutical industry.

In the last couple of decades, some out-of-the-box physicians started to realize the flaws withT4-only therapy. Hence, they started to prescribe desiccated thyroid preparations. In addition, alternative medicine practitioners have been prescribing these preparations all along.

These pills contain both T4 and T3 in the proportions present normally in pig and human thyroids: A ratio of 4:1. Each one grain is equal to 60 or 65 mg (milligram). It contains about 38 mcg (microgram) of T4 and 9 mcg (microgram) of T3.

As these pills come from the *whole* thyroid gland, they contain all of the ingredients of the thyroid gland. That's why they also contain MIT (Monoiodotyrosine) and DIT (Diiodotyrosine), in addition to T3 and T4. Please refer to Chapter 4, for more information on MIT and DIT.

In addition, they also contain calcitonin, which is a hormone produced by the thyroid gland. Calcitonin is primarily involved with calcium and bone metabolism. In this way, these pills provide you with all of the thyroid hormones that your own thyroid gland normally produces.

Dessicated thyroid is available as Thyroid in Canada, Thyroid-S in Thailand, Thyroid Extract in Australia, Thyreogland in Germany, and Whole Thyroid in New Zealand.

2. Levothyroxine Plus Liothyronine

Some people do not like the *idea* of getting pills from animals. Or they may be allergic to pig or beef or one of the Dessicated Thyroid pills. In these patients, I prescribe both T4 (Levothyroxine, brand Synthroid, Levoxyl, Unithroid, Levothroid) and T3 (Liothyronine, brand Cytomel). I give T4 and T3 in a ratio of about 4:1 to *mimic* the normal daily production of these hormones.

For example, I may give a patient a daily dose of T4 (Levothyroxine) as 100 mcg and T3 (Liothyronine) as 25 mcg.

Sometimes, I use a ratio of T4 to T3 as 3:1, especially in my obese individuals in whom T4 to T3 conversion is often impaired.

3. Customized T4 and T3 Combination Preparation from a Compounding Pharmacy:

Sometimes, using T4 (Levothyroxine) and T3 (Liothyronine) in the correct ratio can be tricky. Why? Because T3 (Liothyronine) comes only in three strengths: 5, 25 and 50 microgram tablets. T4 (Levothyroxine) is available in many strengths, but still the precise amount for an individual may fall in between the two strengths. Then, it becomes difficult to precisely *titrate* the dose.

Some individuals are very sensitive to slight changes in T3 or T4. In these patients, I sometimes resort to compounding pharmacies, which can compound T4/T3 combination according to the formula I write down.

Note:
There is a synthetic product, in which there is a combination of T4 and T3 in a ratio of 4:1. Its generic name is Liotrix and brand name is Thyrolar.

However, since 2007, this product is on a long-term back order due to some manufacturing changes, per its manufacturer, Forest Pharmaceuticals. For most hypothyroid patients, it used to work very well. The only problem was that it had to be kept in a refrigerator.

Beware:

Due to pressure from patients, some physicians may reluctantly prescribe T3. However, many are afraid to use T3, as they do not have in-depth knowledge about the intricacies of T3, T4 and TSH, as I outlined earlier in the book. Therefore, they will use only a small dose of T3 such as 5 mcg of Cytomel. Consequently, you will continue to suffer from hypothyroidism. Then, you may think that even T3 did not work for you. You think there must be something really wrong with you.

Case Study No: 4

A 68 year old Caucasian female was referred to me by her cardiologist for the treatment of hypothyroidism.

She was diagnosed with hypothyroidism at age 28. Initially, her internist placed her on a daily dose of Armour Thyroid 4 grains, which is equal to 240 mg. She felt good at this dose.

About 13 years ago, her gastroenterologist took over her thyroid management and gradually lowered the dose of Armour Thyroid to 1 grain a day. She gained 45 Lbs. in 3 months and slept about 16 hours a day. She started experiencing a lot of fatigue. Then, she decided to see an internist who had a special interest in thyroid management. This physician put her on Thyrolar, 2 grains twice a day. Thyrolar is a synthetic drug combination of T3 and T4, compared to Armour Thyroid, which is natural and comes from pig and beef.

She lost about 30 Lbs. and got her energy back. Then, this physician retired.

Then, she went to see another internist, who switched her from Thyrolar to Synthroid 200 mcg a day and added Cytomel in a small dose of 5 mcg a day.

She again started feeling tired. In addition, she also developed irregular heart beat, called atrial fibrillation, for which she started seeing a cardiologist, who started to lower her dose of Synthroid as "her T4 was too high and TSH was too low." She became more lethargic and gained about 30 lbs. in one year.

Then, she saw an endocrinologist, who advised her to decrease Synthroid from 200 mcg (microgram) per day to 150 mcg per day and stop taking Cytomel. On this regimen, her heart rate dropped and averaged about 35 beats/minute. She felt exhausted. Her endocrinologist told her to continue the same dose of Synthroid and to stay away from Cytomel. She got dissatisfied with her endocrinologist. Subsequently, her cardiologist increased her dose of Synthroid to 175 mcg a day, added Cytomel 12.5 mcg every other day and sent her to see me for a second endocrine consultation.

When I saw her, she complained of severe fatigue, difficulty losing weight and excessive hair loss. She was on Synthroid 175 mcg a day and Cytomel 12.5 mcg every other day. In addition, she was on Premarin (estrogen), Furosemide (a water pill), and Singulair (asthma medication). Interestingly, she noticed that she did not have atrial fibrillation on the days that she took Cytomel, but atrial fibrillation would recur on the days she did *not* take Cytomel.

Her laboratory tests, ordered by her cardiologist were as follows:

- **TSH** = less than 0.02 mIU/L ((normal range, 0.4 - 4)
- **Total T4** = 15.9 mcg/dL (normal range, 5-12),
- **Total T3** = 233 ng/dL(normal range, 82 - 179.)

I assessed her Total T4 and Total T3 to be high due to elevated TBG (Thyroid Binding Globulin), as she was on estrogen. (see chapter 1 for excess TBG).

Although she was on both Synthroid and Cytomel, the *ratio* was *not* correct. She was on too small a dose of T3 and too high a dose of T4. That's why she was still suffering from hypothyroidism due to low T3 in the peripheral tissues. Meanwhile, her TSH was low because of too high of a dose of T4, which her pituitary was appropriately responding to. *In other words, her pituitary gland was healthy but the rest of her body, including muscles and heart was not.* As usual, her physician was treating TSH and not the patient.

I increased her T3 to 25 mcg every day instead of every other day, and reduced her T4 to 100 mcg per day. On this regimen, she immediately started feeling better.

At Three Months:

Her laboratory test was as follows:
- **Free T3** = 3.1 pg/mL
- **Free T4** = 0.9 ng/dL
- **TSH** = 0.04 mIU/L.

She felt energetic and episodes of her atrial fibrillation had markedly decreased.

At Six Months:

Her laboratory test was as follows:
- **Free T3** = 2.5 pg/mL
- **Free T4** = 0.9 ng/dL
- **TSH** = 0.11 mIU/L.

She reported that her atrial fibrillation would occur only at about 3-4 am, lasting for about 60 minutes, and disappear after she took her dose of thyroid hormones. T3 does not last in the body as long as T4 does. I assessed that her T3 level came down after about 18 hours and may have been causing atrial fibrillation.

Therefore, I switched her to T4 = 45 mcg + T3 = 15 mcg twice a day, from a compounding pharmacy.

At Ten Months:

Her laboratory test was as follows:
- **Free T3** = 2.9 pg/mL
- **Free T4** = 0.8 ng/dL
- **TSH** = 0.05 mIU/L.

She felt great. Episodes of atrial fibrillation had reduced in frequency.

At Sixteen Months:

Her laboratory test was as follows:
- **Free T3** = 4.0 pg/mL
- **Free T4** = 1.0 ng/dL
- **TSH** = 0.03 mIU/L.

She was thrilled to report that she no longer has atrial fibrillation. She is thrilled to share her experience with other patients.

****

Can low T3 cause atrial fibrillation?

The usual medical thinking is that T3 increases heart rate and may cause atrial fibrillation. However, this may *not* be entirely true. The above-mentioned case study clearly indicates that the *reverse* may be true in some patients: low T3 may be associated with atrial fibrillation.

There is an exciting research article published in 2005 in the *Journal of Cardiothoracic Vascular Anesthesia*, in which researchers from Finland found a strong relationship between low T3 and the risk of developing atrial fibrillation (1).

When To Take Thyroid Hormone?

All thyroid hormone pills should be taken on an empty stomach, in the morning. Don't eat for about one hour. This enhances the absorption of the thyroid hormone.

If T3 is a large dose, such as more than 15 mcg (microgram), it should be split into two doses: One dose in the morning and a second dose before lunch.

Drug Interactions

There is drug-to-drug interaction between Thyroid hormones and several commonly prescribed drugs.

Estrogen such as
Oral Contraceptives
Oral estrogen pills (PREMARIN, ESTRACE etc.)

Estrogen increases TGB (Thyroid-Binding-Globulin). Consequently, your blood level of total T4 and total T3 gets elevated, but Free T4 and Free T3 levels are usually normal. Transdermal estrogen such as estrogen patches and skin creams do not seem to have this effect.

****

Warfarin (COUMADIN):
The addition of thyroid hormone makes you more *sensitive* to warfarin, the dose of which needs to be decreased. Test for clotting, such as INR, should be done more frequently until you have achieved a stable dose of warfarin.

****

The following agents can *decrease* the absorption of thyroid hormone. Therefore, these agents should be taken at least **four** hours after thyroid hormone:

Calcium
Iron
Antacids
sucralfate (CARAFATE)
cholestyramine (QUESTRAN, LOCHOLEST)
cholesevelam (WELCHOL)
raloxifene (EVISTA)
Grapefruit juice
Ciprofloxacin and similar antibiotics

****

The following drugs can *decrease* the level of thyroid hormone in the blood. Consequently, your dose of thyroid hormone may need to be titrated upwards.

Anti-epilepsy drugs such as
phenobarbital (LUMINAL),
phenytoin (DILANTIN)
carbamazepine (TEGRETOL),
oxcarbazepine (TRILEPTAL),
primidone (MYSOLINE),

Anti-depressant drugs such as
sertraline (ZOLOFT)

Some Antibiotics such as
rifampin (RIFADIN),
rifabutin (MYCOBUTIN),
nevirapine (VIRAMUNE)
efavirenz (SUSTIVA).

****

Allergy To Dessicated Thyroid

If you develop allergy to any drug, you may be allergic to the drug (active ingredient) or the filler (inactive ingredient).
In the case of Dessicated Thyroid, you may be allergic to pig, beef, or the fillers.

Armour thyroid was reformulated in 2009, and corn-starch was added as a filler. Since then, a lot of individuals have reported having allergic reactions.

If you develop an allergic reaction to one of the Dessicated Thyroid pills, and you are *not* allergic to pig or beef, then it is likely that you may be allergic to one of the fillers. Various Dessicated Thyroid preparations have various fillers in them. Therefore, it is worthwhile to switch to a different Dessicated Thyroid preparation.

Sometimes, you may need to switch from Dessicated Thyroid to synthetic T4 (Levothyroxine, brand Synthroid, Levoxyl, Unithroid, Levothroid) and T3 (Liothyronine, brand Cytomel), Or you may decide to go to a compounding pharmacy, with a customized ratio of T4 and T3, written by your physician.

****

Case Study NO: 5

A 52 year old Caucasian female consulted me for thyroid nodule. She also had Hashimoto's thyroiditis. I placed her on Armour thyroid 15 mg a day. She felt great on it, but 3 weeks later, developed an allergic reaction, causing swelling of her face. I advised her to stop Armour thyroid, and to take Benadryl. After a few days, she was back to normal. At this point, I started her on Nature-throid 16.25 mg a day, which she tolerated well. She did not develop any allergic reaction to Nature-throid.

****

Monitoring the Dose

I closely monitor the dose of thyroid hormones, according to the following parameters:

- Are the symptoms of hypothyroidism improving?

- Is Free T3 in the upper half of the normal range or not?
- Is TSH getting in the range of 0.4 - 2.0 mIU/L?
- Is Free T4 in the low normal range?
- Is the patient developing any symptoms due to too much thyroid hormone?

Generally, I see my hypothyroid patients every 3-4 months and check their blood test for Free T3, Free T4 and TSH. Accordingly, I may make necessary adjustments in the dose of thyroid medicine.

In general, your dose of thyroid hormone is *dependent* on your weight. If you gain weight, you need a higher dose of thyroid hormones. The converse is also true: if you lose weight, you need a smaller dose.

Special Situations

A. In older individuals as well as anyone with atrial fibrillation or heart disease, I start out on a small dose of T3 and T4, especially T3 and increase it gradually: *Low and Slow approach*. I take this conservative approach because T3 may increase their heart rate, which is undesirable in these patients.

I usually start out with only a small amount of T3 (Liothyronine) such as 5 -10 microgram a day and for the rest, I use T4 Levothyroxine.

B. In older individuals who have undergone complete thyroid removal by surgery due to thyroid cancer, I use only a small amount of T3 (Liothyronine) such as 5-10 microgram a day and a relatively large dose of T4 (Levothyroxine), because I want to suppress their TSH to prevent the recurrence of thyroid cancer, especially if their thyroid cancer was the *aggressive* type. T4 is actually very effective in suppressing TSH, as a relatively high level of T4 leads to high T3 formation inside the pituitary gland, which suppresses TSH production.

C. Some individuals need a higher dose of T3 (Liothyronine) to get rid of their symptoms of hypothyroidism. Their T3 level in the blood may even get slightly above the normal range.

It is okay if they do not have a history of heart disease, atrial fibrillation or osteoporosis, and as long as they do not develop palpitations of the heart, and are taking a large dose of Vitamin D to prevent osteoporosis.

D. **During pregnancy,** your dose of thyroid hormone generally goes up, mostly due to weight gain. Therefore, I see my patients every two month during pregnancy. In the second half of the pregnancy, I also check their blood for TG antibodies, TPO antibodies and TSI (Thyroid Stimulating immunoglobulin). If positive, there is a risk of autoimmune thyroid disease in the fetus as these antibodies do cross the placenta.

After delivery, your dose of thyroid hormone comes down as you shed the pounds gained during pregnancy.

Keep A Broader Perspective

As I mentioned earlier, when treating hypothyroid patients, I keep a broader perspective. For example, most hypothyroid patients are low in Vitamin B12 and iron as well. Almost everyone is low in vitamin D. Most consume more food than their body needs. Almost everyone suffers from the stress of daily living. Therefore, I keep a broader perspective and treat all of these factors, in addition to appropriate treatment with T3 and T4.

Treat The Underlying Cause

In addition to treating the symptoms of hypothyroidism, I treat the underlying root cause of hypothyroidism. Only then, can one hope to cure hypothyroidism. In the following chapters, I elaborate on my strategy to treat these root causes of hypothyroidism.

References:

1. Kokkonen L, Majahalme S, Kööbi T, Virtanen V, Salmi J, Huhtala H, Tarkka M, Mustonen J. Atrial fibrillation in elderly patients after cardiac surgery: postoperative hemodynamics and low postoperative serum triiodothyronine. *J Cardiothorac Vasc Anesth.* 2005 Apr;19(2):182-7

Chapter **10**

How to Cure Hashimoto's Thyroiditis (Autoimmune Thyroiditis)

As you recall from Chapter 6, Hashimoto's Thyroiditis is a form of autoimmune thyroiditis, which is accompanied with a goiter. The other form of autoimmune thyroiditis is called atrophic thyroiditis, which is *not* accompanied with a goiter.

In autoimmune thyroiditis, your immune system starts to attack your own thyroid cells. But why? In other words, what causes autoimmune thyroiditis? If you ask your physician, the likely response will be, "Oh, we know genetics is a factor. Besides that, we don't know much about it."

Even if you do a search on the internet or read textbooks on Hashimoto's thyroiditis, you won't find any more information in this regard.

It is true that autoimmune diseases, including Hashimoto's thyroiditis, tend to congregate in families. You're at a high risk of developing an autoimmune disease if you have a family history of an autoimmune disease. For example, your mother may have Hashimoto's Thyroiditis or Graves' Disease, while your sister may have Asthma or Crohns' Disease. Your brother may have Celiac disease.

Here is a list of various autoimmune diseases.

- Autoimmune Thyroid Disease, which can either cause you to have a low level of thyroid hormone (Autoimmune Thyroiditis) or a high level of thyroid hormone (Graves' Disease).
- Gluten Sensitivity/Celiac Disease
- Vitamin B12 Deficiency
- Pernicious Anemia
- Asthma
- Eczema
- Alopecia areata
- Ulcerative Colitis
- Crohns' Disease
- Type 1 Diabetes
- Vitiligo
- Psoriasis
- Adrenal Insufficiency/Addison's disease
- Multiple Sclerosis (M.S.)
- Chronic rheumatologic conditions such as Rheumatoid Arthritis, Fibromyalgia, Systemic Lupus Erythematosis (commonly known as Lupus) and Ankylosing Spondylitis.

What Really Causes Autoimmue Thyroiditis?

MY OWN CLINICAL RESEARCH

Not every genetically predisposed individual (not even twins) develops an autoimmune disease. We cannot do anything about genetics anyway. Are there some other factors responsible for autoimmune dysfunction and can they be treated? As an endocrinologist, I was curious about these questions. What I discovered is amazing!

In all of my patients with autoimmune diseases, including Autoimmune thyroiditis, I discovered the following **three** factors play a crucial role in causing an autoimmune disease. What is even more exciting is that all of these factors are treatable.

Treatable Factors That Cause Autoimmune Thyroiditis

1. Worrying.
2. High Carbohydrate diet.
3. Vitamin D deficiency.

1. Worrying

I found that each and every one of my patients with Autoimmune thyroiditis (as well as Graves' disease and other autoimmune diseases) *worries* a lot. How can worrying cause autoimmune dysfunction?

Normally, your immune system is designed to deal with threats, let's say an invading virus. When faced with an army of viruses, your immune system recognizes these invading biologic agents as foreign and recruits an army of its own white cells, called lymphocytes. Think of these activated lymphocytes as soldiers called to duty. A battle takes place between the army of the viruses and your activated lymphocytes. If you win, you get over the viral illness. Then, these activated lymphocytes are sent back to the barracks. No more threat, no more need for the army of the activated lymphocytes.

Well, when you worry excessively, you are basically afraid that something bad may happen. In other words, your mind perceives a threat, *albeit* a virtual threat. The immune system reacts to the threat: virtual or real - It doesn't matter. An army of the activated lymphocytes is recruited. Think of the activated lymphocytes as *hyped* up soldiers looking for the enemy, but there is *no* enemy. The threat is virtual, but they have to attack someone. So they start to attack your body's own cells, such as thyroid cells.

Think of the thyroid cells as *innocent* bystanders, who get scared and start to run after seeing soldiers carrying guns. This simply energizes the soldiers. They mistakenly believe they have found the enemy and start to attack and destroy the thyroid cells.

As thyroid cells start to die out, thyroid hormone production starts to decrease. Normally, your pituitary gland increases its production of TSH in response to low thyroid hormones as I described earlier in the book.

However, the pituitary gland is usually unable to increase its production of TSH in these individuals. Why? Because there is an increased production of cortisol in these stressed out individuals, which has a *negative* effect on TSH production. Consequently, your TSH level does not rise, but remains normal, while your thyroid hormone production goes down, at least in the early stages of the disease. Due to this process, early hypothyroidism remains undiagnosed, because your physician is trained to diagnose hypothyroidism only if TSH is elevated.

Upon your insistence, a conscientious physician may decide to do a test for thyroid antibodies, which would be elevated. Then you are told, "Well, you have Hashimoto's thyroiditis, but there's nothing I can offer at this time. We have to wait until your TSH gets elevated." With this mindset, a lot of *precious* time is wasted, while your activated lymphocytes continue to destroy your thyroid cells. Ultimately, there is a *significant* decline in your thyroid hormone production due to a lot of damage to your thyroid gland. At this point, your TSH production is so high that it erodes through the negative effect of cortisol, and your TSH level finally gets elevated.

As you will learn, we can do a lot to stop the immune-attack on the thyroid gland. The sooner we implement this strategy to treat the autoimmune process, the better the results.

Elevated TSH over-stimulates the remaining thyroid cells to produce extra quantities of thyroid hormone. An analogy would be your boss asking you to take on an extra load of work after a number of workers have been laid off. Just like an extra work load would create stress for you, elevated TSH creates stress for the remaining thyroid cells. Under stress, these cells try to proliferate more and may form *nodules* within the thyroid glands. But even then, thyroid hormone production continues to fall down.

Thyroid nodules make physicians in the U.S.A. very nervous. Why? Because they're afraid of being sued if they miss a cancerous thyroid nodule. To put things in perspective, the odds of having a cancerous nodule are extremely small: 90 - 95% of nodules are non-cancerous. In addition, thyroid cancer is a very slow growing cancer and has a great prognosis in the vast majority of cases.

The news that you have a thyroid nodule makes you more worried. All the information you get from your physician as well as the internet, *turbo* charges your pre-existing anxiety. You may go through a couple of Fine-Needle Aspiration Biopsies. Even the benign results of these biopsies may not provide you and your physician with enough *comfort* level. You might decide to have the nodule/nodules surgically removed. Then you end up having half (or sometimes even more) of your thyroid gland surgically removed.

Please note that thyroid nodules also develop in patients without Autoimmune thyroiditis. How you deal with a thyroid nodule is ultimately your choice in consultation with your physician.

After thyroid surgery for a thyroid nodule, your thyroid hormone production goes down even further. Often, your physician does not even put you on thyroid hormone, while you continue to suffer from hypothyroidism as well as Autoimmune thyroiditis. **Remember, surgery does not cure your autoimmune dysfunction.**

You may even worry more, as now you have a lot of symptoms due to inadequately treated hypothyroidism, and no one seems to know how to fix your thyroid problem.

2. High Carbohydrate Diet

Extensive scientific studies have clearly established that diet plays an important role in the *causation* and *progression* of autoimmune diseases. But how?

Certain genetically predisposed individuals are not able to digest starches and sugars properly. The partially digested starches and sugars provide fertile grounds for bacteria and yeast to thrive in the intestines, causing "bacterial overgrowth." The byproducts of these micro-organisms cause inflammation of the intestinal walls, making them more permeable. Large molecules of partially digested food can then leak into the blood stream. This is called **Leaky Gut Syndrome**, which in turn, activates your immune system.

The activated lymphocytes then start to attack various organs in the body, giving rise to a variety of clinical symptoms. In the case of Autoimmune thyroiditis, these activated lymphocytes attack and destroy your thyroid cells.

Therefore, starches and sugars play an important role in causing and perpetuating autoimmune diseases including Autoimmune thyroiditis.

3. Vitamin D Deficiency

Vitamin D is actually not a vitamin, but a hormone. Vitamin D is produced in the skin from 7-dehydrocholesterol (pro-vitamin D3) which is derived from cholesterol. Here is evidence that cholesterol is not all bad, contrary to what most people think these days. The fact is that cholesterol is a precursor for most hormones in your body.

Type B Ultraviolet rays (UVB) from the sun act on pro-vitamin D3 and convert it into pre-vitamin D3, which is then converted into vitamin D3. Medically speaking, we call it cholecalciferol. Vitamin D3 then leaves the skin and gets into the blood stream where it is carried on a special protein called a vitamin D-binding protein.

Through blood circulation, vitamin D3 reaches various organs in the body. In the liver, vitamin D3 undergoes a slight change in its chemical structure. At that point, it is called 25, hydroxy cholecalciferol or 25 (OH) Vitamin D3 (or calcifediol). It is then carried through the blood stream to the kidneys where it goes through another change in its chemical structure. At that point, it is called 1,25 dihydroxy cholecalciferol or 1,25 (OH)2 vitamin D3 (or calcitriol). This is the active form of vitamin D. It gets in the blood stream and goes to various parts of the body and exerts its actions

Vitamin D plays an important role in the normal functioning of the immune system. Therefore, a deficiency of vitamin D can lead to a malfunction of the immune system. There is *mounting* scientific evidence that links vitamin D-deficiency to autoimmune diseases including Hashimoto's thyroiditis.

A well designed, case-control study was published in January 2013, in *Endocrine Practice*, the official journal of the American Association of Clinical Endocrinologists. This study (1) showed a clear relationship between vitamin D deficiency and Hashimoto's thyroiditis.

In this study, researchers investigated vitamin D level in three groups: those with long-standing Hashimoto's thyroiditis and hypothyroidism, those with newly diagnosed Hashimoto's thyroiditis and a control group without Hashimoto's thyroiditis. They measured 25 (OH) vitamin D level, thyroid antibodies and thyroid size with ultrasound. The findings were remarkable. Vitamin D deficiency had a correlation with thyroid antibodies, thyroid size and duration of Hashimoto's thyroiditis.

In other words, those with newly diagnosed Hashimoto's thyroiditis had a vitamin D level lower than those without Hashimoto's thyroiditis. However, those with longstanding Hashimoto's thyroiditis and hypothyroidism had a vitamin D level even lower than those who were newly diagnosed with Hashimoto's thyroiditis. The plausible explanation: Vitamin D deficiency may *not* only cause Hashimoto's thyroiditis, but also perpetuate it.

In another study (2), low vitamin D (level less than 30 ng/ml) was present in 92% of patients with Hashimoto's thyroiditis compared with 63% of healthy controls This study was published in 2011 in *Thyroid*, official journal of the American thyroid Association.

In another remarkable study (3), published in 2012 in the *Journal of Pediatric Endocrinology and Metabolism,* researchers compared vitamin D level in children who were newly diagnosed with Hashimoto's thyroiditis with a control group of children without Hashimoto's thyroiditis. They found that vitamin D deficiency was present in 73% of children with Hashimoto's thyroiditis compared to only 18% of the control group

There is strong scientific evidence to *incriminate* low vitamin D as an important factor in the causation of other autoimmune diseases such as rheumatoid arthritis (4), lupus (5,6), fibromyalgia (6), multiple sclerosis (7,8), and Type 1 diabetes (9). In an experimental study from UCLA School of Medicine, vitamin D deficiency was found to cause Graves' Disease (10).

My own clinical experience at the Jamila Diabetes and Endocrine Medical Center demonstrates vitamin D level to be low in every patient with autoimmune diseases, including patients with Autoimmune thyroiditis.

My Strategy to Cure Autoimmune Thyroiditis

Based on the evidence I just presented, I developed a clinical approach to cure autoimmune dysfunction, including Hashimoto's thyroiditis. This approach consists of three components:

- Freedom from worrying
- A special low carbohydrate diet
- Vitamin D 3 supplementation

I discuss this 3-component approach in length with my patients who suffer from Hashimoto's Thyroiditis and other autoimmune dysfunctions. I have seen some great results in those patients who put this approach into practice. Nothing can be more gratifying to see this kind of results in my patients.

I have picked two actual cases of severe Hashimoto's thyroiditis from my clinical practice, to demonstrate that Hashimoto's thyroiditis, even in its most severe form, can indeed be cured.

Case Study NO: 6

A 44 year old Caucasian female was diagnosed with Hypothyroidism and placed on Levothyroxine 100 mcg daily, by her primary care physician.

Five Months later:
TSH was low as 0.05 mIU/L (reference range, 0.40-4.50)
Free T4 = 1.3 ng/dL (reference range, 0.8-1.8)
Total T3 = 85 ng/dL (reference range, 76-181)
TPO antibodies = 970 IU/ml (reference range, <35)
Tg antibodies = 31 IU/ml (reference range,<20)

Her TPO antibodies were markedly high. Clearly, she was suffering from Hashimoto's thyroiditis. On her own, she saw an endocrinologist, who told her that *nothing* can be done about her Hashimoto's Thyroiditis.

She was *not* satisfied with this answer. She decided to seek a second opinion and came to see me. At that time, She was on Vitamin D3 as 2000 IU a day, and her TPO antibodies were markedly elevated at **>1000** IU/ml.

I discussed my Stress Management Approach, special low CHO diet and increased her Vitamin D3 to 6000 IU a day. Instead of Levothyroxine, I placed her on T3+ T4 combination from a compounding pharmacy and gradually increased it to T3 =15 mcg + T4 = 50 mcg a day. She has stayed on this dose for most of her clinical course under my care.

Here are her progress-notes.

At Eight Months:

TPO antibodies came down to **111** (reference range, <35)
Tg antibodies were negative (reference range < 20 IU/ml) and have remained negative for the rest of her clinical course.
25 OH vitamin D = 62 ng/ml
TSH = 2.33 mIU/L
Free T4 = 1.0 ng/dL
Free T3 = 2.7 pg/ml (2.3-4.2)

At Thirty Four Months:

TPO antibodies were down to **64** (reference range, <35)
25 OH vitamin D = 73 ng/ml
TSH = 2.25 mIU/L
Free T4 = 0.8 ng/dL
Free T3 = 2.8 pg/ml (2.3-4.2)

At Forty Months:

TPO antibodies were down to **26** (reference range, <35). In other words, her Hashimoto's thyroiditis had resolved.
25 OH vitamin D = 77 ng/ml
TSH = 0.86 mIU/L
Free T4 = 0.8 ng/dL
Free T3 = 2.6 pg/ml (2.3-4.2)

At Forty Seven Months:

TPO antibodies were 19, which meant her Hashimoto's thyroiditis continues to be resolved.

25 OH vitamin D = 120 ng/ml
TSH = 1.91 mIU/L
Free T4 = 0.8 ng/dl
Free T3 = 3.1 pg/ml (2.3-4.2)

Despite a vitamin D level above the normal limit of 100 ng/ml, her blood Calcium level was perfectly normal at 8.8 mg/dL. In other words, she did *not* have vitamin D toxicity, because the hallmark of vitamin D toxicity is a *high* calcium level in the blood. More on Vitamin D toxicity in Chapter 13.

She feels thrilled to know that her Hashimoto's thyroiditis is cured, and wants to share this important information with other patients who suffer from Hashimoto's thyroiditis.

****

Case Study No: 7

A 51 year old Caucasian male consulted me for fatigue and weight gain. His labs showed:

Free T3 = 1.75 pg/ml (reference range, 3.0 - 4.2)
Free T4 = 0.5 ng/dL (reference range, 0.8 - 1.8)
TSH = 96 mIU/L (reference range, 0.40 - 4.50)
TPO antibodies >1000 IU/ml (reference range, <35)
Tg Antibodies = 28 (reference range, <20)
25 OH vitamin D level = 27ng/ml (reference range, 30 - 100)

I placed him on Synthroid 112 mcg a day and Cytomel 5 mcg a day, vitamin D3 as 8000 IU a day and also discussed my stress management approach.

At Three Months:

Free T3 = 2.96 pg/ml,
Free T4 = 1.1 ng/dL,
TSH = 7.45 mIU/L, and
25 OH vitamin D = 46 ng/ml.

He had lost 7 Lbs. and felt better.

At Six Months:

Free T3 = 3.24 pg/ml
Free T4 = 1.0 ng/dL
TSH = 3.46 mIU/L
25 OH vitamin D = 50 ng/ml

He had lost total of 12 Lbs. Had good energy level. I increased vitamin D dose to 10,000 IU a day.

At Nine Months:

Free T3 = 3.54 pg/ml
Free T4 = 1.3 ng/dL
TSH = 2.0 mIU/L
25 OH vitamin D = 72 ng/ml
TPO antibodies were down to **71** from >1000 IU/ml
Tg Antibodies were < 20 and have stayed <20 for the rest of the clinical course.

At Twenty Four Months:

Free T3 = 3.4 pg/ml
Free T4 = 0.9 ng/dL
TSH = 8.17 mIU/L
25 OH vitamin D = 66 ng/ml
TPO antibodies =178

I switched him from Synthroid and Cytomel to Armour Thyroid 90 mg a day.

At Thirty Two Months:

Free T3 = 3.4 pg/ml
Free T4 = 0.9 ng/dL
TSH = 4.88 mIU/L
25 OH vitamin D = 51 ng/ml

TPO antibodies = 78

Free T3 = 3.6 pg/ml
Free T4 = 0.8 ng/dL
TSH = 3.5 mIU/L
25 OH vitamin D = 60 ng/ml
TPO antibodies = 33, which meant his Hashimoto's thyroiditis had resolved.

At Fifty One Months:

Free T3 = 4.3 pg/ml
Free T4 = 0.9 ng/dL
TSH = 3.29 mIU/L
25 OH vitamin D = 81 ng/ml
TPO antibodies = 30, which meant his Hashimoto's thyroiditis continues to be resolved.

He has stayed on the same dose of Armour Thyroid for more than 2 years.

Initially, his LDL was elevated as 153 mg/dl. Within 3 months of the treatment of hypothyroidism, his LDL came down to 108 and has stayed under 120 over the course of more than 4 years of follow-up. He has not been on any cholesterol-lowering drugs.

Lessons to Learn:

With proper treatment, Hashimoto's thyroiditis can be cured.

By curing Hashimoto's thyroiditis, you stop further damage to the thyroid gland. Then, you don't need to keep increasing the dose of thyroid hormone with the passage of time.

Once autoimmune dysfunction is cured, patients do not develop other manifestations of autoimmune dysfunction.

Some patients with Hashimoto's thyroiditis have elevation in both TPO and TG antibodies, while others have elevation in only one type of antibodies and not the other.

Hypothyroidism is one common cause of elevated LDL cholesterol. Effective treatment of hypothyroidism alone often brings LDL level into a good range.

****

I elaborate on my special approach to cure Hashimoto's thyroiditis, in the next three chapters.

References:

1. Bozkurt NC, Karbek B, Ucan B, Sahin M, Cakal E, Ozbek M, Delibasi T. The Association Between Severity of Vitamin D Deficiency and Hashimoto's Thyroiditis. *Endocr Pract.* 2013 Jan 21:1-14

2. Tamer G, Arik S, Tamer I, Coksert D. Relative vitamin D insufficiency in Hashimoto's thyroiditis. *Thyroid.* 2011 Aug;21(8):891-6

3. Camurdan OM, Döğer E, Bideci A, Celik N, Cinaz P. Vitamin D status in children with Hashimoto thyroiditis. *J Pediatr Endocrinol Metab.* 2012;25(5-6):467-70

4. Merlino LA, Curtis J, Mikuls TR et al. Vitamin D intake is inversely associated with rheumatoid arthritis: results from the Iowa Women's Health Study. *Arthritis Rheum* 2004;50:72-77

5. Kamen DL, Cooper GS, Bouali H, et al. Vitamin D deficiency in systemic lupus erythematosus. *Autoimmune Rev* 2006;5:114-117

6. Huisman AM, White KP, Algra A, et al. Vitamin D levels in women with systemic lupus erythematosus and fibromyalgia. *J Rheumatol* 2001;28:2535-2539.

7. Hayes CE. Vitamin D. a natural inhibitor of multiple sclerosis. *Proc Nutr Soc.* 2000;59(4):531-535.

8. Raghuwanshi A, Joshi SS, Christakos S. Vitamin D and multiple sclerosis. *J Cell Biochem.*2008;105(2):338-343.

9. Hypponen E, Laara E, Reunanen A, et al. Intake of vitamin D and risk of Type 1 diabetes: a birth-cohort study. *Lancet* 2001;358:1500-1503.

10. Misharin A, Hewison M et al. Vitamin D deficiency modulates Graves' hyperthyroidism induced in BALB/c mice by thyrotropin receptor immunization. *Endocrinology.* 2009, 150(2):1051-1060.

Chapter **11**

Freedom From Worrying

What I discovered is that patients with Hashimoto's thyroiditis and other autoimmune diseases *worry* a lot about every little thing. Often, they are *afraid* of this or that.

When you worry, your body thinks that it is under attack. Therefore, your immune system gets into a high alert state to fight off the offending agent, but there is no one to fight off! Confused, it starts to attack its own organs, causing a variety of diseases. If it attacks the thyroid gland, you can develop Graves' Disease (which results in hyperthyroidism) or Hashimoto's Thyroiditis (which can result in hypothyroidism).

Why Do We Worry?

Use logic and you realize the underlying cause of "worrying" is <u>fear</u>.

Fear comes in many forms. Some examples:

1. Fear of the Future

You may be afraid something *bad* may happen in the *future*, based upon your *past* experience or the experience of others that you have heard about through chatting, the news media, internet, books or knowledge of history.
You *do not* want it to happen to you ever, because it was (or could be) so painful. The mere thought that it may happen *triggers* a wave of fear and anxiety in you. This leads to "What If Syndrome" or "What May Syndrome" or "What Will I Do Syndrome."

Here are some examples:

- What if I have another attack of asthma, colitis or a migraine headache?
- What if Wall Street takes a nose-dive again?
- What if I get stung by a bee again?
- What if I miss my important meeting?
- What if I develop diabetes and die a miserable death like my mother?
- What happens if global warming continues?
- What happens if some bad people come into power?
- What if there is a severe shortage of my thyroid medication, insulin or water supply?
- What will I do if run out of my retirement money?
- What will I do if my mother/father/children are not around any more?
- What will I do if someone breaks into my house in the middle of the night?
- What will I do if I have no money, no insurance, no friends?
- What will I do if someone tries to rob me or rape me?
- What if my boyfriend/girlfriend cheats on me?

2. Fear of Losing

Often, you are afraid to lose what you have. For example:

- Fear of losing your job, business, money, stocks, retirement.
- Fear of losing your spouse, parents, children, siblings, friends, pets.
- Fear of losing your looks.
- Fear of losing your house, car, jewelry, photo-albums.
- Fear of losing your respect, credibility, position, reputation.
- Fear of losing your professional license.

- Fear of losing your power.
- Fear of losing your composure, self-control.
- Fear of losing your No. 1 spot.
- Fear of losing your health.
- Fear of losing your independent living.
- Fear of losing your life.
- Fear of losing your religion, culture, country.
- Fear of losing elections.
- Fear of losing planet earth.

3. Fear of Failure

You may be afraid you won't be able to live up to expectations. For example:

- Fear of failing as a good mother/ father.
- Fear of failing as a good child.
- Fear of failing as a good brother/ sister.
- Fear of failing as a good friend.
- Fear of failing as a good teacher/ student.
- Fear of failing as a good boss /employee.
- Fear of failing as a good doctor, teacher, lawyer, etc.
- Fear of failing as a good guru, enlightened person, yoga instructor.
- Fear of failing as a good driver, pilot or captain of the boat.
- Fear of failing as a patriot, soldier or general.
- Fear of failing as a good citizen, journalist, moral person.
- Fear of failing as a good social, religious or political leader.
- Fear of failing as a nice person, who keeps his/her appointment, commitments, promises, wedding vows.

4. Fear of Social Situations

You may be fearful of humiliation and criticism. For example:

- Fear of rejection, social outcast.
- Fear of embarrassment.
- Fear of shame.
- Fear of insults.
- Fear of being late.
- Fear of premature ejaculation, sexual performance or impotence.

5. Fear of Punishment And Sufferings

Fear also arises when you are afraid of punishment and painful sufferings. For example:

- Fear of being caught: with a prostitute, cheating, bribing, stealing, swindling, having sex, being nude, watching pornography, masturbating, living as an illegal immigrant, driving without a license, practicing without a license.
- Fear of monetary penalty.
- Fear of social boycott.
- Fear of imprisonment.
- Fear of torture.
- Fear of deportation, poverty and its associated sufferings.
- Fear of sufferings from disease and disability.

6. Fear of Lack Of Control/Vulnerability

You may be afraid of being vulnerable. Here are some examples:

- Fear of the unknown.
- Fear of the outcome.
- Fear of unpreparedness.
- Fear of lack of knowledge.

ULTIMATE FREEDOM FROM FEAR

In order to be free of fear, first you need to find out what is the root cause of fear, instead of running away from fear and finding a quick fix. The quick fix approach will be superficial, a band-aid that won't work effectively in the long run. That's why anti-anxiety medications may provide you with temporary relief of symptoms arising out of fear, but they do not get rid of fear at its roots. Many other techniques to conquer your fear may suppress your fear for a while, but deep down you continue to be fearful.

So, what's the root cause of fear?

The Root Cause Of Fear

Use common sense, and you will see that fear is an emotion, triggered by a "frightening thought." The emotion of fear then influences your thought process, which becomes more frightful. Then, it generates more emotions of fear. Thus, a vicious cycle sets in: thoughts generate fear and fear generates more thoughts.

This vicious cycle can induce some neurochemical changes in your brain as well as release of the hormones adrenaline and cortisol from the adrenal glands. All of these chemical changes give rise to manifestations of fear, which range from insomnia, anxiety and phobias to panic attacks, allergies and autoimmune disorders.

What Is The Basis Of Thoughts?

It is pretty clear that thoughts give rise to fear. Where do thoughts come from? While pondering over this question one day, I made a simple, yet profound observation. We humans, always think in terms of a language. For example, if you know English and no other language, you will always think in English, not in Chinese, French or Hindi. Just observe it right now, yourself.

In order to think, you need to know a language. Therefore, language is the basis of thoughts.

What Is The Basis Of Language?

Obviously, the next question is where does the language come from? You are not born with it, right? You learn it as you grow up in a society. You learn it from your parents, teachers, siblings, friends and various tools such as books, electronic devices and sometimes, certain other techniques.

What Is A Language?

Let's use common sense and explore what is a language. It is a means to communicate with each other. A language is comprised of words, right? And each word has a <u>concept</u> attached to it. In reality, every word is a sound. For example, listen to a language you don't know. All you will hear is sounds, sounds that make no sense. In order to make sense, you need to know the concepts attached to the sounds. In this way, we can say that a word consists of a <u>sound</u> and an attached <u>concept</u>. Even written language has <u>concepts</u> attached to words. Even Sign language has <u>concepts</u> attached to signs.

What Is The Basis Of Concepts?

Let's use common sense and find out where concepts come from. Concepts are the creation of a society, aren't they? When you grow up in a society, your parents teach you the language of that society. They utter a sound and point to a person or some object. They keep repeating it until you make a *connection* between that sound and the person or object. For example: As a baby, you hear the sound Mama as your mother points a finger towards herself. After a lot of repetition, you make a connection between the sound and the person. She is no longer another life form, but Mama. She provides you with food, comfort and warmth. You get *attached* to her. Later, she provides you with toys, gifts, friends, cupcakes, cookies, money and so on. You get more and more attached to "your Mama."

As you grow up in a society, you are *bombarded* with concepts that the society has created, such as the concepts of success, failure, achievement, money, fame, desirable, undesirable, morality, etiquette, responsibility, culture, customs, religion, nationality, past, future, security. Based on these concepts, certain thoughts may arise, such as thoughts of losing, being a failure, an outcast, punishment, suffering, the future, insecurity, etc. All of these thoughts create a huge amount of fear.

Sooner or later, you are introduced to the concept of death. Then a thought runs through your head - What if my Mama dies? This triggers a wave of fear and anxiety throughout your body.

As you grow up in a society, you also acquire a lot of information, all of which is based on language. In other words, you need a language to understand any information. Your society provides you with this information, usually in the form of the news media, books, internet, etc. In this way, you acquire a lot of information about some dreadful event that happened hundreds *if* not thousands of miles away. Perhaps, that tragic incident happened years or even centuries ago, before you were even born. Based on all of this fearful information in your head, some new thoughts arise. "What if it happens to me?" "What will I do?" All of these thoughts then trigger a lot of fear in you.

Who Is Thinking?

If you pay attention, you realize it is always "I" who is afraid of this or that. It is the "I" who is thinking. Therefore, it is the "I" who is at the <u>root</u> of all of the fear. Who is this "I"? We need to figure this out, if we truly want to be free of fear.

The Virtual "I"

Who is this "I" that is thinking and is fearful? You may reply, "Oh! It's me." Really?

Let's take a look at this "I". Can you show me where is it? It's in your head, isn't it? It's an abstraction, an illusion, a phantom. It is a *virtual* entity in your head that *steals* your identity. It is not the "true" you at all. Why do I say that? Because you are not born with this. In order to know your "True, Original Self," observe little babies, just a day or so old. I had the opportunity to be in charge of a well-baby nursery in my early career as a doctor and observed about sixty babies every day. Later, I had the wonderful experience of having my own baby.

When you observe little babies, you see that as soon as their basic physical needs are met (ie. a full stomach, a clean diaper and a warm blanket), they are *joyful* from within! They *smile* and go to sleep. They have no *past* or *future*. They are *not* worried if mom will be around for the next feed. If they did, they wouldn't be able to go to sleep. They don't think. Hence, there is no concept, no future and consequently, no *fear* and no *worries*. That's why they have no problem going to sleep. They are so *vulnerable*, but *fear* remains miles away. There is a total *lack of control,* but *no fear* whatsoever.

Once their stomach is full, they *don't* want any more food. If you were to force more food than they need, they would regurgitate. They eat to satisfy their hunger and that's all. *Wanting more* does not exist and that's why they are so *content.* You could feed them breast milk, cow's milk or formula. To them, it doesn't matter as long as it agrees with their stomach and satisfies their hunger.

They don't say "I don't like your milk, Mom. I like formula milk better." You won't hear, "Mom, you wrapped me in a pink blanket with butterflies on it. I'm a boy. Therefore, I need a blue blanket with pictures of dinosaurs on it."

They are joyful just looking around. They truly *live in the moment.* They do it spontaneously without making an effort to live in the Now.

Why do I say newborn babies don't think? Because, you always think in terms of a language. Newborns know *no* language. Hence, they don't think. They also have no concepts. Why? Because concepts arise out of language. No language - no concepts.

Newborn babies don't like or dislike someone because of their color, religion, nationality or wealth. That's because they have not acquired any *concepts* about religion, nationality, history or money. *Concepts* do not exist at all. *Likes and dislikes* do not exist. There are no *preferences or judgments.* No *embarrassment or shame.*

No fear, no anger, no hate, no wanting more, no prejudices... Just pure joy, contentment and peace. Every moment is *fresh, pristine* and *new. This is the True Human Nature.* I like to call it the "True Self," the self that you and I and everyone else on the planet is born with.

Now let's see what happens to this fearless, joyful and peaceful baby.

The Acquired Self

Gradually, another self develops as you grow up in a society. This, we can call the *Acquired Self.* You acquire it as a result of *psychosocial conditioning*, from your parents, your school and then, your society in general.

As you grow, this Acquired Self gets bigger and bigger. It gets in the driver seat, pushing the True Self onto the passenger side and later, into the back seat and eventually, into the trunk.

As a grown up, all you see is this Acquired Self. You identify with this Acquired Self. *That's who you think you are.* This becomes the virtual "I" sitting in your head. Your identity gets *hijacked* by the Acquired Self. Instead of seeing the hijacker for what it is, you think that's who you are. How ironic!

This Acquired Self is the basis for all of your stress, including worries. It reacts to outside triggers, which it calls stressors and blames them for your stress. In fact, it is the Acquired Self who reacts to triggers and creates stress for you. In this way, the source of all stress actually resides insides you. It is good to know this very basic fact. Why? Because if the source of stress is inside you, so is the solution.

This Acquired Self torments you and creates stress even when there is no stressful situation. It conveniently creates *hypothetical* situations (the What If Syndrome) to make you fearful. I like to call it a *monster*, as it is quite frightening and appears strong, but in the end, it is really virtual.

Sadly, you don't even have a clue what's going on, because you completely identify with the Acquired Self, the mastermind behind all of your stress. You could call it the *enemy within*.

Unfortunately, you're completely out of touch with your True Self, the source of true joy, contentment and inner peace. In the total grip of the monstrous Acquired Self, you suffer and suffer and create stress not only for yourself, but for others as well.

The Composition Of Your Acquired Self

At the core of your Acquired Self is the virtual, conceptual "I" you *mistakenly* think you are. Around this "I," there are layers and layers of concepts, information and knowledge, downloaded into your growing Acquired Self. Some examples: My parents, My teachers, My friends, My school, My career, My goals, My car, My house, My beauty, My jewelry, My ancestors, My accomplishments, My culture, My town, My country, My religion, My past, My future.

The Making Of The Virtual "I"

Where does the virtual "I" come from? It is actually a concept that gets downloaded into your head.

It starts from home. Your parents carefully select a label for you. They call it your name, which is basically a sound. Your parents utter this sound as they point towards you. After doing it repeatedly, they finally succeed in drilling into your head that you are indeed Peter, Lisa or Susan. At the same time, they also drill in the concepts of Mama and Dada.

As you grow up in a society, you acquire more and more concepts, which circle around the concept of "I," just like the layers of an onion.

How Your Acquired Self Creates Fear For You

Once your Acquired Self *steals* your identity, it *runs* your life. Then, you experience life through the *filters* created by your Acquired Self. These filters come from concepts, knowledge, information and experiences. The experiences can be your own as well as the experiences of others (virtual experiences for you), in the form of stories and opinions you saw in newspapers, books, magazines, TV or the internet or heard from friends and family.

Basically, your Acquired Self wants to live a very secure life. It wants security. Why? Because it is *inherently* insecure. It is *not* real. It is virtual, a phantom, an illusion, but it thinks it is real and it wants to live forever. Pretty crazy, isn't it?

In order to be safe, your Acquired Self *interprets* every experience (real experience or virtual experience. It doesn't matter) based on the information stored in it and judges the experience to be good or bad, which triggers an emotion, good or bad. Then, it *stores* the entire experience along with the triggered emotion into your *memory* box, where it stays *alive*, even years later. This is how your mind creates your *memories* or the past.

Experiences which are labeled good, your Acquired Self wants *more* of and the ones labeled bad, it wants to *run* away from. This is the basis of psychological *attachment* and *avoidance*.

Your Acquired Self gets very *attached* to good experiences, such as praise and validation, which provides a *temporary* relief from its insecurity. That's why your Acquired Self gets attached to the <u>concepts</u> of *money, power* and *success*, all of which bring it praise and validation. With money and power, it can acquire *possessions,* which enhances its *ego* and provides *temporary* validation and relief from insecurity.

Your Acquired Self is often very attached to the concept of beauty. Why? Because it provides praise, validation and temporary relief from insecurity. However, you end up spending a lot of time and money to look beautiful. You become a frequent visitor to beauty parlors, shopping malls and may even see a plastic surgeon to enhance/preserve your looks. You get stuck with huge bills, which create more stress. Then, one day you may notice wrinkles on your face or excessive hair loss, which may push a *panic* button. In my practice, I have had patients wanting to be seen on an urgent basis because they noticed clumps of hair falling out of their head during their morning shower. They act like it's the end of the world.

Your Acquired Self also gets *praise* from family, friends and fans regarding its success, fame and accomplishments. It wants more and more of these experiences. It also feels *validated* when it is related, bonded or responsible for someone. For example, if you own a pet, it *validates* the existence of you as an owner and provides your Acquired Self a temporary relief from insecurity. That's why it doesn't want to ever *lose* its pets, family, friends and fans. *Even the idea of losing them rips through the paper thin layer of security and stirs up deep-seated, inherent insecurity which triggers a huge amount of fear.*

Your Acquired Self also seeks validation through conceptual identities such as a doctor, lawyer, teacher, political, social or religious leader, movie star, employee of a certain company, citizen of a certain country, member of a certain social, political or religious group, etc. That's why even the thought of losing its virtual identity creates a huge amount of fear. This is why you are so afraid of the possibility of losing your professional license, career, citizenship, elections, etc.

Your Acquired Self does not *ever* want to *lose* anything or anyone that is "Mine." That would mean losing a part of "Mine." How terrible that would be! That's why it is afraid of losing possessions. The more possessions you have as "My, Mine," the more you *fear* losing them and the more you try to protect them. You may end up living in a gated community to protect your belongings. Even news of someone getting robbed creates a lot of fear for you.

In addition, your Acquired Self wants to *avoid* unpleasant experiences, such as failure, punishment, loneliness, humiliation, poverty, aging, disease and death at all costs. *Even the thought of such unpleasant experiences triggers intense fear.*

In order to be secure, your Acquired Self also uses the following strategy. It has been conditioned to *learn* from its past. So it uses its past experiences or even the experiences of others that it has heard about and creates *hypothetical,* frightening situations, which is the basis of "What If, What May Syndrome." Then, it tries to find solutions, which is the basis of "What Will I Do Syndrome."

In reality, those situations don't exist at all. In other words, your Acquired Self is so *insecure* and *afraid* of its own death, that it creates all *possible,* dreadful case scenarios and tries to *figure out* how it can *escape* its death in every possible way. In doing so, it creates tons of *unnecessary* fear for you.

Your Acquired Self also quickly wants to interpret every situation it encounters and every person it meets, based upon stored information. Why? Because it wants to feel secure. Often, it judges a person to be safe or unsafe, based upon their appearance, without even exchanging a word. Often, it doesn't want to take any chances, so it won't interact with anyone it doesn't know.

You may remember "don't talk to strangers" from your childhood. You also want to make sure to download this very important message into the growing Acquired Self of your children. Maybe you read a story about some girl who got abducted by a stranger in a place you know nothing about. It rips through your feeling of security. Ironically, it reinforces your self-fulfilling prophecy of being "fearful of strangers." Obviously, you don't hear or pay attention to the countless safe encounters with strangers.

Your Acquired Self also wants to know everything about the future in order to feel safe. Otherwise, it suffers from fear of the unknown.

Your Acquired Self is very afraid of your death, because it fears its own death. Therefore, any thought about death triggers a huge amount of fear.

Be The Master Of Your Acquired Self, Not Its Slave

The root cause of your fear and all other stress actually resides inside you - your Acquired Self. Therefore, the solution must also reside inside you.

In summary, your Acquired Self is the virtual, conceptual "I" you *mistakenly* think you are. It's consists of "My name, My personality, My beliefs, My past, My future, My parents, My children, My teachers, My friends, My students, My school, My career, My goals, My accomplishments, My failures, My culture, My town, My country, My religion, etc. It is a virtual *entity* sitting inside you, but it is not the *true* you. It *steals* your identity. It controls your *thoughts*, *emotions* and *actions*.

The Acquired Self is the basis of the "Busy Mind," a *constant* stream of thoughts. Then, thoughts *provoke* emotions and emotions *taint* your thoughts. A vicious cycle of thought-emotion-thought sets in. This is the basis of worrying, anxiety, anger, frustrations, hate, love, revenge, jealousy, guilt, sadness, depression, selfishness, greed, ego, self-righteousness, expectations, judging, hypocrisy, embarrassment and shame. Then, *actions* arise out of these thoughts and emotions, which often cause stress for you and others. The actions may be verbal, written or physical.

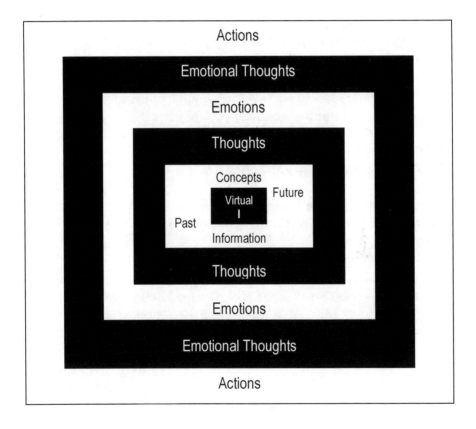

The Acquired Self

How To Rise Above Your Acquired Self

First of all, you have to see your Acquired Self as separate from you. Only then, can you see it for what it is. However, if you continue to *identify* with your Acquired Self, you can *never* see its true colors. As long as you and your Acquired Self are *stuck* together, obviously you can *never* be free of it.

In order to *free* yourself from your Acquired Self, you have to see it in action. When you're in the grip of your Acquired Self, you *immediately* react to *triggers*. We can call it auto-pilot mode. These automatic reactions often cause more stress for you and others. Later on, when you come to your senses, you often *regret* what you said or did.

1. Don't React Immediately!

The *first step* to *separate* yourself from your Acquired Self is to *not* let it automatically control your actions. Stop for a moment and *pause* before you *react* to what you read, hear or watch.

2. Shift Your Awareness/Attention To The Now

Shift your attention to the *Now*. What is Now? Now is *not* what is in your head, but what is in front of your eyes. It is your field of awareness.

Pause for a moment right now and pay attention to what you see, what you hear, what you smell, what you taste and what you touch. Don't think, just observe. Experience what's in your field of awareness.

In general, when we see, we only pay attention to objects without paying any attention to the *space* in which everything is. Without space, there would be no objects. So when you see objects, also be aware of the space which gives rise to all objects.

In the same way, when you listen, also pay attention to the *silence*, without which there would be no sound.

Use your eyes and ears and be aware of space, *silence* and *stillness*, which gives rise to all objects, events and sounds.

In addition to your outer field of awareness, you also have an *inner field of awareness*. This inner field of awareness is your *Original Self*.

It is vibrant, full of immense energy, joy and inner peace. No words can accurately describe it... But it can be felt. It is Real and not a concept. That's why your Acquired Self, which consists of concepts, cannot understand it. You can feel your inner field of awareness simply by calming your busy mind and taking your attention inside you.

In fact, your outer field of awareness is an extension of your inner field of awareness. It is <u>one</u> field of awareness... And that is what the Now is! I made this arbitrary distinction of inner and outer field of awareness just to communicate with you. That's all!

Practice to be aware of the Now around you and inside you. Then, you can easily *shift* your attention to the *Now* as soon as you realize your thoughts and emotions have taken over you.

The moment you switch your attention to the Now, you are free of your thoughts and their associated emotions. In other words, you are free of your Acquired Self. *Instantaneously,* you will feel *relief* from fear or any other stressful emotion. That's how powerful this seemingly simple step is. A moment later, your attention may again be *sucked* up by thoughts and emotion. Simply keep shifting your attention/awareness into the Now.

Your Acquired Self needs your *attention* to thrive. That's why it *sucks* up your attention/awareness most of the time. However, you have the power to *switch* gears and *divert* your attention/awareness to the Now. Without your attention/awareness, your Acquired Self can no longer survive. As long as your attention/awareness is in the Now, you are free of the Acquired Self.

Remember this phrase: <u>Keep your mind where your body is</u>.

While fully aware of the Now, feel and watch the drama your Acquired Self creates. Don't run away from it. After a little while, it will settle down.

Example:

You're stuck in traffic on your way to the airport. You start worrying. "What if I miss my flight and then I'll miss my interview for this job I really want and my best chance to get this dream job will evaporate" and on and on. You get so *fearful* from the drama that your Acquired Self creates, that you may end up having chest pain and find yourself heading to a hospital... Or you can choose to shift your attention from thoughts to the Now: Watch the car in front of you, the cars to each side, the median of the freeway, the electric poles seemingly running backwards, the sky, the clouds, etc. Also pay attention to your breathing, which is a continuous act in the Now. Chances are pretty good that you will arrive at the airport safely, certainly without any fear or high blood pressure. You may or may not be late. If you are late, you will deal with it. Therefore, live in the Now, stay in reality and you won't have any fear.

Caution:

Be careful *not* to confuse *attention* with *concentration*. Attention is simple awareness, that's all! It is there automatically, without any effort. On the other hand, concentration and discipline require a lot of effort and are quite stressful by themselves.

3. Use Logic - Common Sense

Now take the next step: use *logic*, the most wonderful tool we humans have. Why? Because the Acquired Self is always *illogical* and can't stand the blazing *torch* of logic. Therefore, use logic and see the *true colors* of your Acquired Self. See for yourself who is really at the root of fear and all other stress. See how *illogical* your Acquired Self is.

For example, your Acquired Self remains *worried* about the so called future. Use common sense and you'll see whatever your thoughts imply, may or may not happen... But certainly, it's not happening in the Now, in front of your eyes, right? Therefore, it's a phantom, an illusion. How can you really take care of a problem that doesn't even exist? If and when it happens, at "that time, the present moment," you'll be able to take *real* action, instead of the *virtual* action your Acquired Self keeps thinking about, which serves no purpose, but simply generates fear.

Another example: You are in your sixties and doing fine. Then one day, you read in the newspaper that someone important died of cancer. Your Acquired Self triggers a thought... What if I have cancer? This creates another thought of possibly losing your health, autonomy and ultimately dying. This creates a huge amount of fear. You start to feel your heart pounding. You feel uneasiness and anxiety. Then, you start wondering who'll take care of your wife if you die, which further worsens your fear and suddenly, you've got a full fledged panic attack.

Even in the midst of this panic attack, pause, take some deep breaths and start counting your breaths. Look around and see what is actually happening in front of you. Feel the space inside your chest. At the same time, feel the fear, but don't get consumed by it. Fully realize that it is your Acquired Self who is fearful. Your True Self, space, is untouchable. Then, use logic. Ask yourself: Do I have cancer at this moment? Am I losing my autonomy at this moment? You realize you really don't have any problems at this moment. Then, you also clearly see that it is actually your Acquired Self playing tricks with you by creating an imaginary future. The moment you clearly see the Acquired Self for what it is, an entity separate from you, it starts to lose its power over you. Using logic, you also tell your mind: "I will deal with any medical condition, if and when it arises." Make a mental note to discuss it with your doctor on your next visit or even write it down on a piece of paper. You will see fear completely evaporate and you can move on with your everyday life.

In addition, *acknowledge* the basic law of nature: if you are born, then one day you die. There are *no* exceptions to this rule. The Acquired Self however, does not want to die and wishes to live forever. Therefore, it makes death something you must avoid, cheat, conquer, etc. In this way, it creates a lot of *negativity* about death. In the grip of their Acquired Self, many people *worry* about death all their life and then one day they die. How sad!

Stop worrying and start living. You can do it once you are free of your Acquired Self.

Instead of worrying, take action in the present moment. For example, eat right, exercise regularly and take vitamin D every day. There's a good chance you won't develop asthma, colitis, cancer, diabetes, high blood pressure or heart disease. Even if you do develop any medical condition, you will be able to deal with it at that time.

However, if you just keep worrying and don't take any actions, chances are you may develop these diseases. Take real action in the present moment, instead of worrying about the results.

Caution:

Please be aware that I am using the word logic as the simple common sense that every human is born with. I am not using it as intellectualization, rationalization or reasoning.

4. Be Aware Of The Conceptual World We Live In

Have you ever pondered about the world we live in? If you take a fresh, logical look at the human world without preconceived notions, you will find that we live in a *conceptual world*, a *virtual world*, not a real world.

Because everyone around us lives in this collective conceptual, virtual world, we think it is real. Actually, we simply accept it as real and don't even bother investigating whether it is real or not.

For example, let's say you watch the Oscar Awards on TV. Through the goggles of the conditioned mind, (your Acquired Self), you see five actresses nominated for best actress. After a few moments of agony, everyone is told who wins *best actress of the year*. The winner is obviously thrilled and excited, but the other four feel defeated, though they try to force a fake smile. For the winner, the moment has finally arrived, the moment for which she has waited for years. She gets overwhelmed with emotions, but manages to deliver an tearful speech. Then, her moment is over. In a few minutes, it is someone else going through similar emotions.

If you are a serious moviegoer, you have your own opinion as to *"who deserves to be the best actress."* If your choice wins, you are also *thrilled*, but if your choice loses, you will be *disappointed,* sometimes even *angry* and *bitter* about the *unfairness.*

You and the world calls it *entertainment*. You want more of it and the world is well equipped to provide you with more! Over the next several days, you enjoy seeing more and more about the whole event on the internet, TV, newspapers and magazines. You see stories about before and after parties, designer dresses, behind the scenes, etc., etc.

For the next few days, you even talk to your friends about the whole experience and have more fun. Actually, the more you know, the more you can impress your friends and the more special you feel about yourself.

Now, let's look at the whole event from an <u>unconditioned mind - someone without the Acquired Self</u>. Now, what you see is a person coming on stage to receive a shiny peace of metal. Holding that piece of metal in her hands, she gets very emotional, her eyes become tearful and her voice chokes. She says a few words and then everyone starts clapping. Why, you wonder?

Obviously, that piece of metal has a huge *concept* attached to it. The woman appearing on stage is not just a woman, but has a huge *concept* attached to her. The whole drama has a huge *concept* attached to it. *The entire concept reverberates with the concept in your head and in everyone else's head, about Oscars, actresses and actors, movies and the concepts of success, achievement, fame, wealth and glamour.*

In other words, your Acquired Self, the *Baby* Monster, gets fed by the *Papa* Monster of the society! That's why you enjoy it so much. For you and everyone else, it becomes real. Actually, you don't even question whether it is real or not. You watch and talk about it as if it was real.

It is interesting to know that you may be able to see the superficial, virtual nature of the part of the conceptual world that you are not attached to. For example, if you are attached to sports and not to movies, you may *not* be interested in watching the Oscars and may even realize their superficial nature, but you will not miss the Super Bowl, Wimbledon, the World Cup, the Olympics, etc. Each one of these words has huge concepts attached to them - the concepts of *victory, achievement, fame, wealth and glamour.*

If you use logic, you will find that most sports are about a ball that is kicked, thrown, carried and/or hit. The world does not see it that way. It sees these sports as a matter of *fight, victory, achievement, fame, glamour.*

By now, you may understand the virtual, conceptual nature of these events. However, you may say these are occasional events in your life. Well, take a close look at the usual activities of your daily life and you realize that most human activities are in the domain of the conceptual, virtual world.

Here are some examples: (*Let me make it very clear that I am making these observations using simple logic. I am not criticizing, putting down or making fun of any of these concepts. Of course, you don't have to agree with me.*)

The Internet, TV, newspapers and magazines obviously take you into the virtual, conceptual world. Many people start their day reading a newspaper or watching a morning show on TV. They glance through magazines or surf the internet during the day. In the evening, they usually watch TV or surf the internet. Most are hooked on TV or the internet for hours every day.

It's interesting to see some older people complain about young people wasting too much time on the internet, playing video games or texting. Meanwhile, they waste their time reading newspapers, watching TV and talking about politics or religion.

Everything you read in newspapers, magazines and books or watch on TV and the internet is conceptual and virtual, isn't it?

Everything in movies, stage shows, museums and art galleries is conceptual, isn't it? All pictures, paintings and statues are obviously conceptual.

All knowledge, whether history, mathematics, science, arts, geography or business is virtual and conceptual, isn't it? In this way, all of the educational system is conceptual.

Language itself is conceptual. Observe how every word carries a concept with it as we observed earlier in the book.

How about political and social systems? All are conceptual.

How about religious establishments? Those are all conceptual as well.

How about cultures, traditions and values? Those are all conceptual.

In reality, you see mountains, land, buildings, roads, trees, animals, sky, clouds and water. However, on a map you see continents, countries, states, provinces and cities - all conceptual.

How about marriage, romance, engagement, divorce? All are concepts, aren't they?

How about time? Seconds, minutes, hours, days, weeks, months and years. All conceptual. Different cultures have created different calendars.

How about national, religious and cultural holidays? All conceptual.

There are concepts attached to gold, platinum, jewels and diamonds. In fact, these are simply metals and rocks, but there are huge concepts attached to them.

How about money? This concept is so overwhelming that no one ever thinks of it as conceptual.

The Concept Of Money

Almost everyone is in the grip of the concept of money and the economy. For most people, it also creates a lot of worries.

What is the economy? It's a concept isn't it? You can not see the economy. You see currency, which itself is a concept. One Dollar, ten Euros, five Yen, a hundred pesos, fifty Rupees, etc.

If you give a 100 dollar bill to a one year old kid, she will probably put it in her mouth, chew on it or rip it apart. Why? Because she still has no concept of money. However, give the same 100 dollar bill to her when she is a teenager and she will be thrilled to have it. Why? Because by now she has acquired the concept of money. In reality, it is a piece of paper, but of course, there is a concept attached to it.

Everyone wants to make money. Money itself is a concept, but people don't think of it that way. To them money is real. *"You can't do anything without money,"* you may argue, but that still does not make it real. *It may be necessary to some extent, but it is not real. To live in the conceptual world, you need money, but it still does not make it real.*

If you look deeper, you'll find that money is a way for humans to trade with each other. Not too long ago, people also used chickens, eggs, rice, etc. to purchase services from others. Animals don't do it.

Obviously, humans developed the *concept of trading.* The concept of trading came into being when humans started living in communities. For example, "I can exchange my eggs for your wheat." Initially, it served a purpose, but then it took over the human race. The concept of precious metals and money came into being. The more money (or precious metals) they had, the more they could buy. Initially, they bought things of necessity: food items, clothes, houses... But this was not enough. They wanted to acquire more and more. Why? Because society also created other concepts: The concepts of prestige, fame, glamour, enjoyment, entertainment, vacations and power. The more money you have, the more powerful, the more famous and the more prestigious you are. You can also have a high profile life-style.

With money, you can purchase various conceptual objects: the car of your dreams, your dream home, your dream vacation, etc. Money is no longer just a means to buy the things of basic necessities. It is often used to *enhance* your ego, which is part of the Acquired Self.

"Wanting more" is the driving force behind the concept of money. There is never enough of it when you are in the grip of "wanting more." Even a billionaire tries to get more!

What's Wrong With Concepts?

There is nothing inherently wrong with concepts. It is only when they are not treated as concepts, but as reality, that they become problematic and create stress for you and others.

Use logic and you'll realize that *concepts are not reality and reality is not conceptual*... But most of humanity are lost in concepts and believe in them as if they were absolute truth. They get attached to them. They either love them (positive attachment) or hate them (negative attachment). Then, actions arise out of these attachments. Actions arising out of concepts create a huge amount of stress for you as well as everyone else.

Concepts also divide humans into groups. Each group believes their own concepts to be true. This obviously creates *conflict*. One group sees the other group as a *threat* to their collective belief system, which creates collective fear. This often leads to violence, verbal as well as physical and can even lead to battles and wars.

5. Utilize Your Acquired Self To Function In The World

The collective *conceptual* world, which we call the world, downloads a *conceptual* world into everyone's head, which is their Acquired Self. The two worlds are *extensions* of each other and *feed* each other. Basically, it is one big *conceptual* world.

Do Not start to hate your Acquired Self. In fact, your Acquired Self has its relative significance. It is your <u>tool</u> to function in the conceptual world, but obviously it is *not* you. The problem arises when you mistakenly believe your Acquired Self *is* you and you lose your true identity. Then, you are <u>enslaved</u> by your Acquired Self, which creates tons of stress for you and others. On the other hand, you need to *rise* above it and be its <u>master</u>, not its <u>slave</u>.

While interacting in the conceptual world, switch gears and shift some attention to your Acquired Self, but don't get overtaken by it. As soon as you don't need the assistance of your Acquired Self, switch gears and shift your attention to the Now.

In short, you are the *boss* of your attention. You can switch gears to shift your attention between your Acquired Self and the Now, back and forth. In this way, you can *function* in the conceptual world, without being enslaved by your Acquired Self.

6. Stress Free Living

With few exceptions, everyone is consumed by the *conceptual* world in their head, their Acquired Self and the collective, *conceptual* world, which we call the world.

As we observed, the conceptual world is full of stress. That's why people are so stressed out. They don't see any way out. They often *rationalize* their stressful living with statements such as "Oh, stress is part of life. There's nothing you can do about it." Then, they seek refuge in *escapes,* such as drugs, alcohol, partying, vacationing, gambling, etc, which provide only temporary relief and actually add more stress in the long run.

Once you *clearly* realize the *conceptual* nature of the "I" and the *conceptual* nature of the world, you are free of them. With this mental shift, a profound wisdom sinks in and your life becomes *stress free* automatically.

For example, you realize money is a concept. It helps you earn a living in the conceptual world, that's all! You earn money to meet the basic *necessities* of life such as food, shelter, clothing, transportation, etc. However, you clearly see the difference between "necessities" and "wanting." You realize it is the Acquired Self that has a never-ending list of "wanting," which is the basis of greed and lack of contentment.

You also clearly see how the Acquired Self boosts up its ego by pursuing certain respectable professions, by seeking fame, by living in a mansion, by acquiring certain possessions or by living a certain lifestyle. You also see the rat-race everyone is in to make more and more money and how it creates a huge amount of stress in their life.

Once you are free of wanting, greed and ego, you are content with whatever job or business you are in, as long as it provides you with the income to make a basic living. When you are not attached to your house, possessions or lifestyle, you are not worried about losing them.

In the grip of the conceptual world, a lot of people end up doing shady stuff to make more money. Then, they are *afraid* of being caught. Once you are free of greed, you obviously don't get into illegal practices to make more money. Then, you're *not* afraid of being caught, because you're not doing any shady stuff.

In addition, don't seek your *identity* through your profession, certain title or position. Then, you *don't* have thoughts about losing them and worries remains miles away.

As a student or parent of a student, you are no longer in a race to go to a prestigious college. As a student, you figure out what you're good at and pursue that particular field. It may or may not bring you a lot of money, but you are fine with this, because you are free of your Acquired Self and therefore, free of wanting, greed and ego. In this way, you don't have to go through tremendous worries such as "What if I don't get accepted at Harvard?"

You realize <u>rules are concepts</u>, but you also acknowledge their functional value. Therefore, you *follow* traffic rules, you *follow* campus rules, you *pay* your income tax and you *follow* the rules of your profession or business. In this way, you become a perfect law-abiding citizen. You have *nothing* to hide. Then, you have *no* fear of being caught.

You realize <u>marriage is a concept</u>, but you also realize its functional value and *follow* it as a part of living in a society. Free of your Acquired Self, you don't get into the mess of extra-marital affairs, which is the activity of the Acquired Self to enhance its ego or to escape from emotional pains. Obviously, if you don't have any affairs, you don't worry about being caught.

You realize <u>beauty is a concept</u>. Consequently, you *don't* worry if you lose a few hairs, if your hair start turning grey or if a wrinkle or a pimple appears on your face. You don't dye your hair, apply wrinkle cream or see a plastic surgeon. All the *worries* about side-effects of these dyes and creams, the high cost of plastic surgery and its possible side-effects automatically do not arise.

You recognize the conceptual nature of all sports, television shows and stocks Then, you *don't* worry about the loss of your team, the fate of your favorite TV show or the performance of your stocks.

You also realize all political, social and religious groups are virtual. Then, you *don't* take sides and *don't* worry if a certain group or party wins or loses.

You realize that internet, TV, newspapers and magazines keep you *trapped* in the conceptual world. Automatically, you don't spend much time on these activities. Then, you don't hear sensational, horrifying and dreadful news and stay free of unnecessary fear.

Once you realize the universal law of birth and death, you don't worry about death. In order to deal with a disease, you take the appropriate medicine and make necessary changes in your diet and exercise level. You realize you are alive until the moment you die. You realize life is to live and *not* to worry.

In short, *minimize* the conceptual world to bare <u>necessities</u>. In this way, you *free* up a lot of time to spend in the Real world, the Now, where there are no worries or any other type of stress... And it is *not* a boring life. Quite the opposite! Once you are in touch with your True Self, you tap into an *immense* source of <u>joy</u> and <u>inner peace</u>. Then, you have no need to seek thrill, excitement and entertainment.

That's how you live a life that is *joyful, peaceful* and completely *free* of fear as well as any other type of stress.

Chapter **12**

Diet for Patients With Hashimoto's Thyroiditis And Hypothyroidism

I recommend the following diet to my patients with Hashimoto's Thyroiditis and Hypothyroidism. This diet is not only appropriate to treat autoimmune dysfunction, but is also helpful to reduce weight. Remember, obesity is another common cause of hypothyroidism.

WHAT NOT TO EAT

1. No processed food.

No canned foods, snack bars, or pre-cooked dinners. Have fresh foods, real foods and organic foods. The true nutritional value of a food (compared to what is written on the food label) is lost when it is processed, stored or frozen.

Try to grow your own vegetables and fruits. In addition, use a local farmer's market to buy fruits and vegetables. Remember, if a fruit or vegetable has traveled hundreds, if not thousands of miles, it has lost its true nutritional value.

2. Eliminate Starches.

Starches are refined carbohydrates. What is a carbohydrate? In chemical terms, a carbohydrate consists of carbon, hydrogen and oxygen atoms.

As a dietary source, carbohydrates are divided into three types:

A. Monosaccharides, which consists of only one type of simple sugar, such as glucose or fructose. A monosaccharide does not require any further breakdown in the intestines before its absorption into the blood.

B. Disaccharides, which consists of two molecules of monosaccharide bonded together. For example, table sugar (sucrose) consists of glucose and fructose. Milk sugar (lactose) consists of glucose and galactose. A disaccharide requires further breakdown in the intestines before it can be absorbed into the blood. For example, sucrase, an enzyme in the intestinal wall, breaks down sucrose into glucose and fructose. Lactase, another enzyme in the intestinal wall, breaks down lactose into glucose and galactose.

C. Polysaccharides, which consist of hundreds to thousands of glucose molecules bonded together. During normal digestion, these polysaccharides are broken down into glucose, which is then absorbed into circulation. Digestion of polysaccharides is a complex process, which requires several digestive enzymes, including maltase in the small intestines.

A lot of individuals with Hashimoto's Thyroiditis cannot properly digest polysaccharides due to deficiency of specific enzymes in the intestines. Partially digested polysaccharides become a great food for bacteria and yeast to grow, which leads to bacterial overgrowth and Leaky Gut Syndrome (discussed in Chapter 10).

The main polysaccharides in our diets are starches. Therefore, eliminate all starches from your diet. Starches include wheat, rice, oats, barley, rye, corn, potatoes, sweet potatoes and yams.

There is another polysaccharide in our diet called cellulose, which cannot be broken down in human intestines. Therefore, it does not become food for bacteria. Cellulose is our dietary fiber, an important ingredient for our health. It prevents rapid absorption of glucose, lowers cholesterol and forms bulk for stools, which prevents constipation.

It is interesting to note that in nature, plants contain carbohydrates as starch, cellulose and simple sugar, mainly fructose. After a plant is harvested, it goes through processing which gets rid of cellulose and what is left behind is starch. Therefore, we refer to starches as refined carbohydrates.

Some individuals with Hashimoto's Thyroiditis even develop loss of the intestinal villi, which are finger-like projections on the intestinal surface that are extremely important for digestion and absorption of polysaccharides. This is what we call Celiac disease or Gluten Sensitivity. There is a blood test to diagnose Celiac disease. The blood test aims to detect several special antibodies, called anti-tissue transglutaminase antibodies (tTGA) or anti-endomysium antibodies (EMA). Consider having this test done. If the test for Celiac disease is positive, then you should stay on a Gluten-free diet for the rest of your life. A Gluten-free diet means to eliminate all wheat, barley, oats and rye from your diet. You need to read labels carefully.

3. Say No to Sugar, Sugar Substitutes and Sugar Alcohols, but Yes to Honey

Say goodbye to sugar, even brown sugar and sugar-containing food items. Why? Sugar causes Leaky Gut Syndrome. This is how: During digestion, each sugar molecule has to be broken down into glucose and fructose by an enzyme called sucrase before it can be absorbed from the intestines into the blood. A lot of individuals with Hashimoto's Thyroiditis do not have enough sucrase to digest sugar. Undigested sugar then serves as fertile ground for bacterial overgrowth in the intestine, which can lead to Leaky Gut Syndrome. As a result, there is unnecessary stimulation of the immune system, as I explained earlier.

You can use honey as a sweetener, because each honey molecule consists of only glucose. It does not require any breaking down in the intestines before its absorption into the blood.

Avoid artificial sweeteners such as Sucralose (Splenda), Saccharin (SugarTwin, Sweet'N Low), Aspartame (Equal, NutraSweet), Acesulfame (Sunett, Sweet One) and Neotame.

Also beware of sugar alcohols such as Sorbitol, Mannitol, Xylitol, Lactitol, Maltitol, Erythritol, Isomalt, Hydrogenated starch hydrolysates (HSH).

These artificial sweeteners are widely used in processed foods, including sodas, powdered drink mixes, chocolate, cookies, cakes, chewing gum and candies. These products are typically marketed as sugar-free and low calorie, which obviously has great appeal to the general public.

As a general rule of thumb, stay away from all processed food items. These are NOT natural, regardless of what they claim. These are synthetic substances that may have started out from a natural substance, but the final product is far from anything that exists in nature. For example sucralose (in Splenda) is made when sugar is treated with trityl chloride, acetic anhydride, hydrogen chlorine, thionyl chloride and methanol in the presence of dimethylformamide, 4-methylmorpholine, toluene, methyl isobutyl ketone, acetic acid, benzyltriethlyammonium chloride and sodium methoxide, according to the book, "Sweet Deception." This processing obviously makes sucralose unlike anything found in nature.

Artificial sweeteners and sugar alcohols can give rise to a number of side-effects, including gas and abdominal cramping. Why? Because these chemicals are usually not absorbed properly and become a fuel for bacterial overgrowth in the intestines. Some even cause neurologic symptoms such as confusion, headaches or dizziness. In addition, there are serious concerns about their long term safety.

Avoid any food item that contains high fructose corn syrup, as it provides fuel for the growth of bacteria in the intestines and contributes to Leaky Gut Syndrome. In addition, consumption of high fructose corn syrup can lead to obesity, diabetes, heart disease and liver damage.

Some common food items you should avoid because they are loaded with starches and sugar or sugar substitutes: These food items are:

- Bread, rice and pasta. Bread includes white bread, whole wheat bread, sourdough bread, French or Italian bread, bagels, croissants, biscuits, hamburger buns, rolls, pita, Indian naans, tortillas, tacos and many more similar bakery products.
- Potato chips, Nachos, French fries.
- Rice including white, brown as well as wild rice.
- Waffles, pies, donuts, pancakes, pastries, cookies, candy and cakes.
- Chocolate, cereals, pizza, chewing gum.

4. No Sodas, No Fruit Juices and No Alcohol.

Do not drink any sodas, even diet versions. Why? Because sodas are loaded with high fructose corn syrup and sugar. Diet sodas use artificial sweeteners and sugar alcohols.

Also avoid fruit juices, because fruit juices from grocery stores contain only a small amount of real juice and a lot of sugar water. Avoid even freshly squeezed, natural juice. Why? Because you end up consuming a high amount of natural sugar, fructose. For example, instead of eating just one whole orange, you will have to use 3-4 oranges to get about a cup of pure orange juice.

Instead of fresh juice, eat two to three Fresh fruit servings per day. Why? Because whole fruits not only contain sugar (fructose), but also the pulp, which slows down the absorption of sugar. That's why there is less of a rise in blood sugar level after eating a whole fruit, as compared to fruit juice, which causes a rapid rise in blood sugar level.

Avoid alcoholic beverages. Why? Because alcohol is a medically well known toxin for the liver, pancreas, brain and nerves. In addition, alcoholic beverages contain carbohydrates and sugars. For example, most beer comes from malted cereal grains, most commonly malted barley and malted wheat.

WHAT TO DRINK?

Water should be your beverage of choice. In a restaurant setting, order water for your drink. Many people order a soda in a restaurant under peer pressure. Remember your body has not changed because you are in a restaurant.

WHAT TO EAT?

1. Vegetables

For clarification, when I use the term vegetables, I refer to the leaf and stem part of the plant, excluding the roots (such as potatoes, sweet potatoes and yam), which are basically starches.

Eat plenty of vegetables. Include vegetables in every meal. They are a great source of vitamins, minerals and fiber. They are bulk forming, fill up your stomach and satisfy your appetite. They also slow down the absorption of sugar from carbohydrates in your diet.

In general, vegetables contain only small amounts of carbohydrates, which is usually fiber. For example, 1/2 cup of cooked spinach contains only 3 gm of carbohydrates, out of which 2 gm is fiber. Spinach, like many other green leafy vegetables, is a great source of Vitamin A, Vitamin K and Manganese.

Use fresh vegetables of the season. Get them from your own vegetable garden or from a farmers' market. Try to steam them or lightly fry in olive oil.

Use raw vegetables in your salads, such as cucumber, bell pepper and tomatoes.

Certain vegetables *may* decrease the synthesis of thyroid hormone in the thyroid gland. Therefore, these vegetables should be used *sparingly* by patients with Hashimoto's Thyroiditis and hypothyroidism. These vegetables are:
Cauliflower, Cabbage, Broccoli, Spinach, Bamboo Shoots, Bok Choy, Brussels Sprouts, Collard Greens and Kale.

2. Fruits

Eat one to two fresh fruits or 1/2 cup per day. Always use fruits which are in season. Either get them from your own fruit trees or from a farmers' market. Avoid fruits and vegetables which have traveled all around the world.

There is tremendous wisdom why certain fruits and vegetables grow in a certain season and climate. We humans may never be able to comprehend this wisdom. Suffice it is to say that if you live in sync with nature, you will avoid a lot of health problems.

For example, nature produces summer fruits for people in a particular area who are also experiencing summer temperatures. Now, you may be in the winter season, but your grocery store is loaded with summer fruits, brought thousand of miles away from the other side of the equator. Without thinking, you grab these produce items as novelty items. Remember fruits and vegetables are just foods, not items for mental entertainment or ego enhancement.

Certain fruits can decrease the synthesis of thyroid hormone. These fruits are Strawberries, Pears and Peaches. Therefore, you should use them in small quantities only.

In general, fruits are a great source of vitamins and minerals, especially potassium. Fruits contain carbohydrates, but they are mainly simple sugars, fructose, which are easily absorbed from the intestines, because they do not require any further breakdown.

Fruits are a great source of antioxidants. In this way, they help to neutralize the damaging effects of free oxygen radicals that are released as a byproduct of the metabolism of food in the cell or when the body is exposed to cigarette smoking or radiation. These free oxygen radicals can damage the structures inside the cell. This is called oxidative stress and it may play a significant role in causing diseases such as cancer and heart disease. Anti-oxidants help to neutralize oxidative stress. Anti-oxidants consists of Beta-carotene, Vitamin A, Vitamin C, Vitamin E, Lutein, Lycopene and Selenium.

Brightly colored fruits are loaded with anti-oxidants. Fruits that are highest in antioxidant contents are pomegranate, blueberries, strawberries, cranberries, cherries, dates, plums, oranges, apples and pineapples.

Fruits are also a good source of fiber, especially avocados, apple, pear, guava, dates, cherimoya, pomegranate, passion fruit, blueberries, blackberries, raspberries, mango, orange, figs and kiwi fruit.

Avocado, guava, dates and cherimoya are a great source of protein. Avocados are also loaded with omega 3 fatty acids, vitamins C and E, carotenoids, selenium, zinc and phytosterols, which help to protect against heart disease and inflammation.

3. Nuts/Seeds

Nuts and seeds are an excellent source of nutrition. They are a great source of Monounsaturated Fatty Acids (MUFA) and omega-3 polyunsaturated fatty acids. Together, these are called the good fats. Why? Because these fats help to increase good (HDL) cholesterol and lower bad (LDL) cholesterol.

Nuts are also a good source of protein, vitamin E (an anti-oxidant) and fiber. They are also low in terms of carbohydrates. For example, 100 gm of almonds provides you with 21 grams of protein, 12 grams of fiber and only 20 grams of carbohydrates. Compare it to 100 grams of Quinoa, which provides you with roughly 13 grams of protein, 6 grams of fiber and 69 grams of carbohydrates.

Nuts are also packed with vitamins and minerals such as magnesium, phosphorus, potassium, selenium, manganese, folate, copper, calcium and zinc. In addition, nuts contain phytosterols, such as flavonoids, proanthocyanidins and phenolic acids.

There is mounting evidence to show that nuts may reduce oxidative stress and inflammation. Clinical studies show that nuts can reduce the risk of heart disease, age-related brain dysfunction and diabetes (1, 2).

Almonds, pine-nuts, pistachios and peanuts contain more protein than other nuts. Macadamias contains the highest amount of monounsaturated fatty acids, followed by hazelnuts, pecans, almonds, cashews, pistachios and Brazil nuts. Walnuts contain the highest amount of polyunsaturated fatty acids, followed by Brazil nuts, pecans, pine nuts, pistachios, peanuts, almonds and cashews.

Nuts also contain a small amount of saturated fat, the so called bad fat. Almonds contain the least amount of saturated fat and Brazil nuts the highest. While all nuts contain some selenium, Brazil nuts have the highest quantities. Selenium is a good antioxidant, helps the immune system and may prevent some cancers.

As discussed earlier, selenium deficiency, in the presence of iodine deficiency may cause hypothyroidism. Therefore, take a *couple* of Brazil nuts a day to make sure a good supply of selenium.

Pine nuts are one of the richest sources of manganese, which is an important co-factor for the anti-oxidant enzyme, superoxide dismutase. Consequently, pine nuts are good anti-oxidants. In addition, pine nuts contain the essential fatty acid pinolenic acid, which works as an appetite-suppressant by triggering the hunger suppressant enzymes, cholecystokinin and glucagon-like peptide-1 (GLP-1) in the small intestine.

Technically, peanuts are not actually nuts but legumes. Dry beans, peas and lentils are some other examples of legumes.

Like nuts, seeds are a good source of protein. For example, 100 grams of seeds will provide you with 30 grams of protein. Seeds are an excellent source of the amino acids tryptophan and glutamate. Tryptophan is converted into serotonin and niacin. Serotonin is an important regulator of our mood. Low serotonin can lead to depression. That's why many modern anti-depressant medications, such as Prozac, Zoloft, Paxil, Celexa and Lexapro act by increasing the level of serotonin in the brain. Glutamate is a precursor for the synthesis of γ-amino butyric acid (GABA), which is an anti-stress neurotransmitter in the brain and can help to reduce your anxiety.

Like nuts, seeds are also loaded with vitamins and minerals. Pumpkin seeds can block the action of an androgen, DHEA (Dehydroepi-androsterone). This may be helpful in preventing prostate and ovarian cancers.

With so many health benefits, I recommend nuts and seeds to my patients with Hashimoto's thyroiditis and Hypothyroidism. However, nuts can cause you to gain weight. Therefore, use nuts in small amounts.

Use raw nuts and seeds. Do not use salted, sugar-coated or chocolate-coated nuts or seeds for obvious reasons.

4. Meats/Poultry/Fish

Eat meats, poultry and fish, including shell fish. These are excellent sources of protein, vitamins, minerals and contain no carbohydrates. For example, 1 oz (28 grams) of cooked Atlantic salmon contains 6 grams of protein, 3 grams of fat, is loaded with Omega 3 fatty acids, and is also a good source of Thiamin, Niacin, Vitamin B6, Phosphorus, Vitamin B12 and Selenium (3).

Red meat is an excellent source of protein, iron and vitamins, especially vitamin B12. For example, 1 oz (28 grams) of ground Beef, (95% lean meat/5% fat, crumbles, cooked, pan-browned, hamburger) contains 8 grams of protein, 2 grams of fat, and No carbohydrates or sugar. It does contain 20 mg of cholesterol which is only 7% of the daily recommended value (4). Compare it to 1 oz (28 grams) of cooked Quinoa which contains only 1 gram of protein, 1 gram of fat and 6 grams of carbohydrates, but no cholesterol (5).

Eat red meat 2 - 3 times per week. Select lean cuts. Avoid processed meats such as cold cuts, salami and hot dogs, as these often contain added sugar and carbohydrates.

Eat Chicken and/or turkey once a day. These are great sources of protein and vitamins.

Eat Fish 1 - 2 times a week. In addition to providing you with protein and vitamins, these are great source of Omega-3 fatty acids, which are good for your cardiovascular health. However, overconsumption of fish can lead to mercury poisoning.

Remember, vitamin B12 is lacking in plants. Therefore, you often become low in vitamin B12 if you are on a vegan OR vegetarian diet.

5. Dairy

Eat a cup of regular, plain yogurt everyday. It is a great source of healthy bacteria for our intestinal health. It is also a good source of protein and calcium as well.

Include a moderate amount of cheeses in your diet. If you are trying to lose weight, then limit the use of cheese.

Drink a cup of milk per day, provided you are not Lactose Intolerant, which is more prevalent in patients with Hashimoto's thyroiditis. If you have Lactose intolerance, you should try Almond milk.

A lot of individuals with lactose intolerance do well on yogurt and cheeses.

6. Eggs

Eggs are a great source of protein, vitamins and minerals, especially Riboflavin, Vitamin B12, Phosphorus and Selenium. Eggs contain no carbohydrates. Therefore, they are a great nutritional source for people with Hashimoto's thyroiditis and Hypothyroidism.

People are overly concerned about the cholesterol content of eggs. Cholesterol is present in the yolk of the egg. If your LDL cholesterol is elevated, then you should use only egg whites.

HOW TO EAT

Eat three regular meals per day. Dinner should be the lightest meal of the day, lunch the heaviest and breakfast the modest meal. Eat dinner at least 3 hours before bedtime.

Avoid snacks, especially when you're watching TV or working on a computer. If you absolutely must have a snack, then try something like nuts, carrot sticks or other raw vegetables.

Get involved in your food. Read labels on food while you are in the grocery store. You'll be surprised how many food items contain sugar, fructose syrup and corn syrup. Avoid these food items.

Try to prepare your meal yourself, at least over the weekend. Avoid buffets! When you opt for a buffet meal, you want to get the most for your buck (after all, you're only human) and you generally end up overeating. Try to eat at home as much as possible. You can find my original recipes in Part 2 of this book.

If you are trying to lose weight, keep a diary of the food you eat. You may be amazed at how much you really eat, contrary to what you thought.

Eat when you are hungry, not because you're sad or on a computer or you have to socialize with family members and friends. *People often eat because of psycho-social reasons.* That's why they continue to gain weight.

Be aware of your eating habits. Eat slowly and enjoy every bite of your meal. Don't watch TV while eating. Many people overeat because they get too involved in watching a TV show or reading a newspaper and don't keep track of their food intake.

Read these recommendations frequently. This will serve as a reminder. Watch your conditioned mind and see how it tries to lure you to eat foods that you know you should not eat. Be aware of the inner voice such as, "Reward yourself. You deserve this bowl of ice-cream. Eat whatever because you're at a party." The inner voice comes from your conditioned mind, which is the basis of your old, bad, illogical eating behavior. You need to rise above it, simply by observing the inner voice, which actually is your enemy in the sense that it sabotages your health.

Practical suggestions for meals

Breakfast:

Egg omelet using 2-3 eggs.

OR

2-4 hard boiled eggs.
1/2 to 1 cup of yogurt.

Lunch / Dinner:

A bowl of vegetable soup
A plate of grilled chicken and fresh garden salad (you may add salad dressing).
A fresh fruit such as a small apple
A handful of nuts.

OR

A bowl of vegetable soup.
A small chicken or turkey or tuna in a lettuce wrap.
A fresh fruit such as a pear.
A handful of nuts.

OR

Grilled vegetables such as bell pepper, zucchini or eggplant, with chicken or turkey strips, stir fried.
A fresh fruit such as grapes.
A handful of nuts.

OR

Grilled Chicken or Steak.
Grilled or steamed vegetables.
A fresh fruit such as melon.
A handful of nuts.

OR

Shrimp on a bed of steamed vegetables.
A fresh fruit such as an orange.
A handful of nuts.

OR

A bowl of soup.
Fish, grilled or baked.
A fresh fruit such as a small apple
A handful of nuts.

ETHNIC FOODS

Chinese

A cup of won ton soup.
Beef or chicken or shrimp, cooked any Chinese style.
A fresh fruit such as a small apple

OR

Mongolian barbeque beef or chicken.
A fresh fruit such as an orange.

Japanese

2-3 sushi. Avoid rice rolls.
Stir fried beef or chicken.
A fresh fruit such as a small apple.

Mexican

A cup of vegetable soup.
A plate of chicken or beef fajitas, without rice or tortilla.
A fresh fruit such as a small apple.

Indian/ Pakistani

Two pieces of Tandoori chicken.
Mixed vegetables.
A fresh fruit such as melon.

OR

Two Seekh Kebobs.
A plate of vegetables such as okra, spinach, or eggplant.
A fresh fruit such as a small mango.

OR

A small portion of chicken or beef or lamb curry, mixed with vegetables. For example, lamb saag or lamb okra or chicken jalfrezi.
A fresh fruit such as an orange.

Middle Eastern

Chicken or beef kebob and salad.
A fresh fruit such as grapes.

OR

Chicken shawarma.
Grilled vegetables.
A fresh fruit such melon.

Greek

Greek salad.
Gyro meat (no fries or rice).
A fresh fruit such as grapes.

Please see page 219 of the book for RECIPES

References:

1. O'Neil, C.E., D.R. Keast, T.A. Nicklas, V.L. Fulgoni, 2011. Nut consumption is associated with decreased health risk factors for cardiovascular disease and metabolic syndrome in U.S. adults: NHANES 1999–2004. Journal of the American College of Nutrition. 30(6):502–510.

2. Carey, A.N., S.M. Poulose, B. Shukitt-Hale, 2012. The beneficial effects of tree nuts on the aging brain. Nutrition and Aging. 1:55–67. DOI 10.3233/NUA-2012-0007.

3.http://nutritiondata.self.com/facts/finfish-and-shellfish-products/4259/2
4. http://nutritiondata.self.com/facts/beef-products/6192/2

5.http://nutritiondata.self.com/facts/cereal-grains-and-pasta/10352/2

Chapter **13**

Vitamin D Supplementation

You may recall from Chapter 10 that Vitamin D plays an important role in the *normal* functioning of the immune system. There is strong scientific evidence to incriminate low vitamin D as an important factor in the causation of autoimmune diseases including Hashimoto's Thyroiditis and Hypothyroidism.

My vast clinical experience at the Jamila Diabetes and Endocrine Medical Center shows Vitamin D to be low in every patient with autoimmune diseases, including patients with Hashimoto's Thyroiditis and Hypothyroidism.

You may wonder, why do I need Vitamin D supplementation? I live in a sunny place, spend at least 15 minutes a day in the sun, drink milk and take a daily multivitamin, which contains 100% of the recommended dose of Vitamin D. Shouldn't I have enough Vitamin D?

A Pandemic Of Vitamin D Deficiency

Believe it or not, we are facing a *pandemic* of vitamin D deficiency! Fifteen years ago, I started investigating vitamin D levels in my patients. To my surprise, the vast majority turned out to be low in vitamin D.

My experience is in line with other researchers. For example, in a study (1) researchers analyzed the data on vitamin D status in the U.S. adult population from the 2000-2004 National Health and Nutrition Examination Survey (NHANES). They were amazed to discover that 50-78% of Americans were *low* in vitamin D. What's alarming is that the situation is getting worse. In a study (2), vitamin D levels in Americans were found to be lower during the 2000-2004 period compared to the 1988-1994 period. Clearly, vitamin D deficiency is getting out of control.

Not only Americans, but people all around the world are suffering from vitamin D deficiency. For example, in a study from the United Kingdom (3), 90% of adults were found to be *low* in vitamin D according to the national representative data collected between 1992 and 2001. In a study from India (4), about 82% of individuals had varying degrees of *low* vitamin D levels. In a study from China (5), researchers assessed vitamin D levels in women in Beijing and Hong Kong. Over 90% of women in both cities were *low* in vitamin D. In another study (6), investigators found that 82% of Japanese men and women were *low* in vitamin D. In a study (7) from Saudi Arabia, all participants were *low* in vitamin D. In a study (8) from Brazil, 100% of men and women were found to be *low* in vitamin D.

Vitamin D deficiency is the true pandemic of our times. It is perhaps more common than any other medical condition at the present time.

It Spares No Age

Infants, children, adults and elderly are all low in Vitamin D. In my extensive clinical experience, it's rare to find someone who has a good level of vitamin D. In my practice, the age of patients range from 15 to 95. I find an overwhelming majority of these patients to be low in vitamin D. Several studies have clearly demonstrated that vitamin D deficiency spans across all age groups.

It Spares No Geographic Location

According to an old paradigm, vitamin D deficiency exists only in northern areas with severe prolonged winters such as Canada, the Northeastern U.S., the U.K. and other northern European countries. However, in reality, vitamin D deficiency is highly prevalent even in sunny, warm places such as the Middle East, India, Pakistan, Brazil, Mexico, New Zealand and Australia. In my own extensive clinical experience in southern California, I have found that most of my patients are low in vitamin D. Vitamin D deficiency is a global phenomenon.

If you live in northern climates, you are more prone to vitamin D deficiency because you can't get enough vitamin D during winter months. In places above 42 degrees North latitude (approximately a line drawn between the northern border of California and Boston), there isn't sufficient solar UVB (Ultra Violet B) energy to form vitamin D in the skin during winter time (from November through February). In far northern latitudes, this decrease in solar energy may last up to 6 months.

In areas below 34 degrees North latitude (approximately a line drawn between Los Angeles and Columbia, North Carolina), there's enough solar UVB energy for skin synthesis of vitamin D throughout the year. *But even in these areas, the sun can't give you vitamin D if you avoid it by using clothing, sun screen lotions or by simply staying out of it.* Therefore, you may live in a sunny place south of 34 degrees latitude, but still be low in vitamin D.

Several clinical studies have shown that vitamin D deficiency is extremely common in the sunny Middle East, primarily because the skin doesn't get enough sun exposure. Due to cultural habits, people avoid the sun and cover most of their body with clothes. This is particularly true in the case of women living in these countries.

It Spares No Race

Fair skin is more efficient in synthesizing vitamin D from sun exposure as compared to dark skin.

However, people with fair skin avoid the sun more than people with dark skin for fear of skin cancer. Even when they go out, they often apply a layer of sunscreen, which prevents vitamin D synthesis. In my extensive clinical experience, I've found people from various racial and ethnic groups to be low in vitamin D.

What Are The Causes For The Pandemic Of Vitamin D Deficiency?

1. Modern Life-Style

Let's take a historic look on vitamin D. It appears that humans started their journey on planet Earth in Africa where there was plenty of sunshine. These early humans covered little, if any, parts of their body. With slow migration northwards over thousands of years, the skin gradually adapted to colder northern climates by reducing the content of its natural sun screen (melanin) and consequently, skin became lighter in color. People with light skin were then able to synthesize enough vitamin D in brief exposures to sunshine.

Vitamin D deficiency is a relatively new phenomenon. Scientists first recognized it in the seventeenth century in the U.K. and other Northern European countries. Interestingly, it coincided with the period of the *Industrial Revolution* when people flocked to big industrial cities such as London and Warsaw and lived in multistoried buildings with narrow, dark alleys. Pollution from coal burning factories created a thick layer of smog. These factors significantly reduced the amount of sun rays reaching Earth in these regions which already had marginal sunshine during long winter periods.

The phenomenon of the Industrial Revolution continued in the newly discovered lands of America and Canada.

In addition, native Africans were enslaved and transported in ships to America over a period of months. Compare this *rapid* migration to the thousands of years it took for early Africans to migrate to Europe, allowing for their skin to adapt to less sunshine. In contrast, this recent migration was extraordinarily rapid, allowing no time for the skin to adapt to conditions of less sunshine. For this reason, African-Americans as a group are particularly low in vitamin D. In recent years, worldwide migration happens at an even faster pace. In a matter of hours, you can migrate from one region of the world to another. That's why people from various parts of Asia and Africa who migrate to the U.K and North America are particularly low in vitamin D.

Now consider another interesting phenomenon. As a result of the *Industrial Revolution*, people with fair skin were able to rapidly migrate to Southern regions with plenty of sunshine. Their skin didn't have time to adapt to these new sunny environments. Therefore, these fair skinned people started developing skin cancer from excessive sun exposure. This led to the development of sunscreen lotions and the drum beat of "avoid the sun!" Even people with dark skin started applying sunscreen lotions under the impression that "it's a healthy habit."

The main reason we're facing a pandemic of vitamin D deficiency is our modern life-style, which minimizes our exposure to the sun. Our technological revolution has dramatically changed lifestyles around the globe. Most people work indoors. They leave their homes early in the morning and return home around sunset or even after dark (especially during winter time). Even at lunch, most people drive to a restaurant or stay inside to eat. Many people spend their lunch break in their office. Over the weekend, we watch TV or surf the internet for entertainment. Teenagers usually stay indoors hooked to a computer or playing video games rather than going outdoors and playing real sports. While shopping, people are mostly indoors thanks to huge grocery stores and shopping malls. Many of the elderly live in assisted living facilities or nursing homes and don't get any sun exposure.

Just observe yourself. How often do you, your family and friends stay indoors while carrying out usual activities of daily living?

2. Sun Phobia

Over the last 30 years or so, sun avoidance has been successfully drilled into the minds of the general public. People are simply scared of the so-called ill-effects of the sun including skin cancer, wrinkles and aging spots. Due to sun phobia, people avoid sun exposure at all costs. When we go outside for even a little while, we make sure to apply sun screen. Parents compulsively apply sunscreen before they allow their children to go outdoors. Many people don't realize that sunscreen also prevents vitamin D synthesis in the skin.

3. Obesity

Vitamin D is fat soluble. Therefore, it gets stored in the fat in your body. In obese individuals, there is excessive storage of vitamin D in fat. Consequently, the circulating level of vitamin D is low in these individuals. Obesity has reached epidemic proportions in the USA and the rest of the world is also catching up in this regard. The epidemic of obesity is contributing to the epidemic of vitamin D deficiency. It's interesting to note that in most cases, obesity is a product of our modern life-style as well.

In a study (9) from City University of New York, researchers looked at the levels of 25 (OH) vitamin D in 12,927 adults 18 years and older participating in National Health and Nutrition Examination Surveys from 2001-2006 in the USA. They found that overweight and obese individuals were 24% and 55%, respectively, less likely to have an adequate level of 25 (OH) vitamin D compared with their normal-weight counterparts.

In one study (10) from Columbia University Medical Center in New York, researchers assessed vitamin D status in 56 obese men and women (body mass index (BMI) > 35 kg/m(2). Serum 25 (OH) vitamin D was low (mean 45 +/- 22 nmol/l) in all individuals. It was inversely associated with BMI. Each BMI increase of 1 kg/m(2) was associated with a 1.3 nmol/l decrease in 25 (OH) vitamin D.

In another study (11) from Columbia University Medical Center in New York, vitamin D level in 236 morbidly obese adolescents being evaluated for bariatric surgery was assessed. The group consisted of 76 boys and 143 girls; 43% Caucasian, 35% Hispanic, and 15% African American). The vast majority, 82%, were found to be low in vitamin D.

4. Medical Illnesses

Malabsorption:

Because vitamin D is fat soluble, vitamin D deficiency can develop in medical conditions that cause malabsorption of fat, such as surgical resection of the small intestine and stomach, chronic pancreatitis, pancreatic surgery, celiac sprue, Crohn's colitis and cystic fibrosis.

Liver and Kidney Diseases:

Vitamin D from the blood is taken up by the liver where it is transformed into 25 (OH) Vitamin D which in the kidneys is further transformed into 1,25 $(OH)_2$ Vitamin D. Therefore, vitamin D deficiency develops in chronic liver disease such as cirrhosis and in chronic kidney disease.

5. Medications

Some medications can further decrease vitamin D level. These medications include: Phenytoin (brand name Dilantin), Phenobarbital, Rifampin, Orlistat (brand names Xenical and Alli), Cholestyramine (brand names Questran, LoCholest and Prevalite) and Steroids

I often see patients who have been on these drugs for a long time, yet they're completely unaware these drugs can rob them of vitamin D. They react with disbelief when I inform them about the relationship between these medications and vitamin D deficiency. "Why didn't my other doctor tell me about it?" is their usual question. Of course, it's your doctor's responsibility to inform you about the side-effects of medicines. Unfortunately, the reality is that some do and some don't.

So educate yourself and be a partner in taking charge of your health. That's why you're reading this book. Nothing can be more rewarding for me than providing you with the information you need to help take care of your vitamin D needs in collaboration with your health care provider.

6. Current Recommendations on Vitamin D Intake are Inadequate

Many people taking vitamins assume that their vitamin D level is okay because the label on their vitamin bottle says it meets 100% of the daily requirements. This misconception is one of the major reasons for vitamin D deficiency among those people who are proactive in taking care of their health.

Vitamin manufacturers follow government guidelines for the daily recommended amounts of various vitamins and minerals. As of 2013, the recommended daily allowance of vitamin D in the USA is: 400 I.U. (International Units) from birth to age 1, then 600 I.U. from age 1 until age 70, and 800 I.U. if you are older than 70.

In various parts of the world, vitamin D dose is also expressed in microgram (mcg) in stead of I.U. Therefore, you need to convert I.U. into micrograms.

Here is the table to convert from I.U. to mcg

400 I.U.	10 mcg.
600 I.U.	15 mcg.
800 I.U.	20 mcg.

Most researchers in the field of vitamin D (myself included) find these recommendations for vitamin D to be inadequate. In a review article (12) published in the *American Journal of Clinical Nutrition*, the authors concluded that for most people, the optimal level of vitamin D is not attainable with the current recommended daily allowances of vitamin D. In March 2007, a number of researchers published an editorial (13) urging a change in the recommendations on daily intake of vitamin D to at least 1700 I.U. in order to obtain a desirable blood concentration of vitamin D.

Based on my vast clinical experience, most people need a much higher dose of vitamin D to obtain an optimal level of vitamin D. In addition, how much vitamin D a person needs is dependent on a number of factors, as you will learn later in this Chapter. Therefore, the optimal dose of vitamin D varies from person to person, and in the same person from summer to winter. Hence, the one-size-fits-all approach is not very scientific.

DIAGNOSIS OF VITAMIN D DEFICIENCY

It's easy to diagnose Vitamin D deficiency: It's a simple blood test. That's all! However, it needs to be the right test and must be interpreted properly! And that's where a lot of problems arise.

What's The Right Test To Diagnose Vitamin D Deficiency And Why?

Laboratories offer two tests to determine Vitamin D level in the blood. In Vitamin D deficiency, one of them is low whereas the other one is often normal. Most physicians don't know the distinction between these two tests and may order the wrong test. Consequently, they may say your Vitamin D level is normal, when it's actually low.

The Correct Blood Test To Evaluate Your Vitamin D Status Is:

25 (OH) Vitamin D (25-Hydroxy Vitamin D)

The other blood test for Vitamin D is 1,25 $(OH)_2$ vitamin D (1,25 dihydroxy vitamin D). *This is the wrong test to diagnose Vitamin D deficiency! Why?*

There are two reasons why 25 (OH) vitamin D and not 1,25 $(OH)_2$ vitamin D is the right test to diagnose Vitamin D deficiency.

Reason 1

25 (OH) vitamin D stays in your blood for a much longer period of time (half life of about 3 weeks) compared to 1,25 $(OH)_2$ vitamin D (half life of about 14 hours). Therefore, 25 (OH) vitamin D more accurately reflects the status of Vitamin D in your body.

Reason 2

As Vitamin D deficiency develops, your body increases the production of parathyroid hormone by the parathyroid glands situated in your neck. Parathyroid hormone increases the conversion of 25 (OH) vitamin D into 1,25 $(OH)_2$ vitamin D. Consequently, 1,25 $(OH)_2$ vitamin D level in the blood will stay in the normal range (and can even be high) even if you're low in 25 (OH) vitamin D.

Watch Out For The So-called Normal Ranges For 25 (OH) Vitamin D

The normal ranges for Vitamin D come from the era when our concern was just to prevent rickets. A small dose of Vitamin D is enough to prevent rickets. Therefore, a level of 25 (OH) vitamin D of 10 ng/ml (25 nmol/L) or above was established as adequate to prevent rickets. That's why many laboratories continue to report 10 ng/ml (25 nmol/L) as the lower limit of the normal range.

However, in recent years our understanding of the effects of Vitamin D has dramatically changed. Now we understand that Vitamin D can do much more than simply prevent rickets. In fact, Vitamin D is crucial for maintaining many vital functions in the body, such as a healthy immune system and a healthy heart. In addition, an adequate level of Vitamin D helps prevent diabetes, osteoporosis and cancer.

To achieve these goals, many experts in the field (myself included) recommend a level of 25 (OH) vitamin D to be at least 30 ng/ml (75 nmol/L) and preferably above 50 ng/ml (125 nmol/L).

Unfortunately, many laboratories continue to report a normal range with the lower limit of 10 ng/ml (25 nmol/L). Now imagine the following scenario: Your 25 (OH) vitamin D level is 19 ng/ml.; Your physician interprets this as normal because it's in the "normal range" provided by the laboratory. However, you are actually quite low in Vitamin D! This happens all too frequently.

Watch Out For The Units Used By The Laboratory

There is another problem that many physicians are unaware of. Different laboratories report Vitamin D level in different units. In the U.S. and around the world, most laboratories report 25 (OH) vitamin D in one of two ways: either as ng/ml or nmol/L.

The conversion factor from ng/ml to nmol/L is about 2.5. For example, if your level is 30 ng/ml, you multiply it by 2.5 and you will get a number of 75 in nmol/L. The lower limit of normal for 25 (OH) vitamin D should be 30 ng/ml or 75 nmol/L.

Now, let's assume that you are fortunate enough to have a physician who keeps up with the latest information and is proactive about Vitamin D supplementation. From attending conferences and reading articles on Vitamin D, your physician may simply remember that the lower limit of normal for 25 (OH) vitamin D is 30 (and that's how most physicians remember - just the numbers, without paying attention to the units).

Here's another treacherous case scenario: Your laboratory reports your 25 (OH) vitamin D to be 40 nmol/L. Your physician simply looks at the number 40 and tells you your Vitamin D is good. In his mind, it's more than 30, so you're fine. In fact, your Vitamin D is low because in reality, a level of 40 nmol/L is equal to 16 ng/ml.!! He totally *forgot* to look closely at the units.

Also, note that the upper limit of normal as reported by many laboratories is also inaccurate. The upper limit of normal should be 100 ng/ml (250 nmol/L).

TREATMENT OF VITAMIN D DEFICIENCY

Most physicians do not know how to properly treat vitamin D deficiency. Why? Because it's not taught during their medical training. Nor do they have much experience in their clinical practice. It's a new field for them.

What amazes me is the advice given in newspaper articles, such as "Experts recommend either 600 units of vitamin D a day or 15 minutes of sunshine a day is enough to get a good level of vitamin D." I believe these recommendations are incorrect.

Why Are Recommendations On The Daily Dose Of Vitamin D Incorrect?

I check vitamin D level in all of my patients. The majority turn out to be low in vitamin D. Many of them take the recommended dose of 600 I.U. of vitamin D a day. Many of them also go out in the sun at least 15 minutes a day in sunny southern California, yet they're still low in vitamin D. Based on this kind of sound clinical evidence, it's clear to me that 600 I.U. of vitamin D a day is insufficient. Fifteen minutes of sunshine a day is also insufficient to get a good level of vitamin D.

Many scientific studies have clearly demonstrated that the current recommended dose of 400-600 I.U. of vitamin D per day is not optimal. An excellent review (1) of these studies was published in the *American Journal of Clinical Nutrition*. The authors concluded that the beneficial blood level of 25 (OH) vitamin D starts at 30 ng/ml (or 75 nmol/L) and these levels of vitamin D can not be achieved in most patients with the daily recommended dose of 400-600 I.U. of vitamin D.

It's also *unscientific* to make general recommendations about how much sun exposure can provide you with enough vitamin D. Why? Because there are many variables that determine vitamin D level in your body including:

1. Latitude
In areas north of 44 degrees N latitude, sun rays are less effective in producing vitamin D in the skin during winter months. The farther north you live, the less effective skin synthesis is from sun exposure.

2. Season
In the same region, the sun is less intense during winter months. Consequently, skin synthesis of vitamin D decreases during wintertime.

3. Age
As you grow older, the skin becomes less efficient in synthesizing vitamin D from sun exposure.

4. Skin Color
The darker your skin, the less efficient it is in forming vitamin D from sun exposure.

5. Sun screens
If you use sunscreen (like most people in the USA), then your skin can't form vitamin D even if you live in a sunny area like Los Angeles or Miami.

6. Lifestyle
Obviously, if you stay out of the sun, you can't form vitamin D in your skin. Many people work indoors and choose leisure activities that are indoors. Similarly, if you cover your entire skin due to cultural reasons (like many women in the Middle-East), you can't form Vitamin D from your skin, even though you live in a sunny place.

With so many *variables* determining vitamin D level, how could "spending 15 minutes a day in the sun" be an accurate recommendation? For example, a New Yorker spending 15 minutes a day in the sun will have a different vitamin D level than a Texan. Even in New York, a person with fair skin will have a different vitamin D level than a person with dark skin. A teenager will have a different level than a grandparent. The same New Yorker will have a different level of vitamin D during summer versus winter. You can see why the "15 minutes of sunshine a day recommendation" is flawed. The "one size fits all" approach doesn't work when you have so many variables!

My Approach To The Treatment Of Vitamin D Deficiency

Over the last thirteen years, I've treated thousands of patients with vitamin D deficiency. Based on my own clinical observations, I've developed a unique, scientific yet practical treatment approach that works well for my patients. My approach to treat vitamin D deficiency is as follows:

1. Assess Vitamin D Status

First of all, I assess and treat every person on an individual basis. I order a 25 (OH) Vitamin D level in the blood to assess vitamin D status. This accurately reflects the impact of all of the *variables* in life style such as geographic location, season, ethnicity, working habits, eating habits, outdoor activities and sunscreen application habits. No guess work. No blind recommendations. To me, this is the most scientific approach in determining one's vitamin D status!

2. Aim For An Optimal Level Of Vitamin D

After the lab test, I discuss the results with my patients.

As I wrote earlier, the level of 25 (OH) vitamin D should be at least 30 ng/ml (75 nmol/L). Now, you may ask, "But what is the optimal level of vitamin D?" Based on my extensive experience, I believe <u>the optimal blood level of 25 (OH) vitamin D to be in the range of 50-100 ng/ml (125-250 nmol/L)</u>. I feel that a vitamin D concentration at this level is important in order to build strong bones, improve immune function, treat aches, pains, chronic fatigue and prevent and treat cancer, heart disease, osteoporosis, tooth fractures, diabetes, high blood pressure, kidney disease and depression.

3. How To Achieve An Optimal Level Of Vitamin D

I discuss with each individual patient various options they can utilize in order to achieve an optimal level of vitamin D.

<u>You can get Vitamin D from Four Sources:</u>

A. Sun exposure
B. Diet
C. Vitamin D supplements
D. Ultraviolet lamps

<u>For an average person, it's impossible to get a good level of vitamin D from sun exposure or diet alone.</u> For example, according to my experience, a Caucasian person needs to be out in the sun in southern California in a bathing suit for approximately two to four hours a day to get a good level of vitamin D. In the case of a person with dark skin, the duration of sun exposure will be about ten hours a day. Now how many people can have that kind of lifestyle year round?

In my extensive experience of diagnosing and treating Vitamin D deficiency, I encountered only one person with a good blood level of 25 (OH) vitamin D (above 50 ng/ml without taking any supplements). She was a lifeguard with fair skin who spent about four hours a day, five days a week in the sun in her bathing suit.

This amount of sun exposure is not only impractical, but also inadvisable. This degree of sun exposure significantly increases your risk for skin cancer, especially if you have fair skin.

Now consider this: One 8 ounce cup of milk has only 100 I.U. of vitamin D. You'd have to drink 20 - 40 cups a day to get a good level of vitamin D. It's not only impractical, but also inadvisable. Imagine all the calories, the amount of LDL (bad) cholesterol and the natural sugar you'd get from such a huge amount of milk.

A serving of cereal fortified with vitamin D has about 40-80 I.U. of vitamin D. You can imagine how much cereal you'd have to eat to get a good level of vitamin D. There are many negative consequences to eating such a large amount of cereal.

From a practical stand point, I recommend taking advantage of three sources of vitamin D: sun, diet and vitamin D supplements. I never resort to ultraviolet lamps, which are expensive and in my experience, unnecessary.

THE THREE SOURCES OF VITAMIN D

1. SUN EXPOSURE

Sun is an excellent source of vitamin D, but it can also cause skin cancer. Various physicians make extreme recommendations on sun exposure, depending upon their specialty. Dermatologists, with their tunnel vision, exaggerate the fear of skin cancer and recommend avoiding the sun as much as possible. And don't forget to put on sunscreen each time you go outside! On the other hand, physicians solely interested in vitamin D, with their tunnel vision, recommend liberal sun exposure and minimize the fear of skin cancer. In my opinion, both have myopic views, which unfortunately, is a basic flaw inherent to modern medicine. Physicians think in the narrow range of their own specialty and don't consider the overall whole outlook for the patient.

Sensible Approach To Sun Exposure

Living in the modern world, you can't obtain a good level of vitamin D simply from sun exposure. However, you should try to get some of your vitamin D from the sun.

The aim should be to get as much sun exposure as you can, without getting a sunburn. How long you can stay in the sun without getting a sunburn depends upon your skin type.

In 1975, Thomas Fitzpatrick, MD, PhD, a Harvard Medical School dermatologist, came up with a classification of skin types, known as "The Fitzpatrick Skin Type Classification System." This system classifies complexions and their tolerance of sunlight.

Type I: Light, pale white. Always burns, never tans

Type II: White, fair. Usually burns, tans with difficulty

Type III: Medium, white to olive. Sometimes mild burn, gradually tans to olive.

Type IV: Olive, moderate brown. Rarely burns, tans with ease to a moderate brown.

Type V: Brown, dark brown. Very rarely burns, tans very easily

Type VI: Black, very dark brown to black. Never burns, tans very easily, deeply pigmented.

Sunbathing

Sunbathing in shorts or a bikini is a great way to get vitamin D as well as other benefits of the sun.

Don't sunbath if you have history of skin cancer or any other disease that can worsen with sun exposure.

There is a lot of confusion about sun exposure, skin cancer and sunscreen usage. Melanoma is the most lethal form of skin cancer, which typically occurs at areas which are not exposed to the sun, such as the upper back and thighs. The melanoma mortality rate has doubled between 1975 and 2010, despite the *rise* in the use of sunscreens during this time. Most authorities agree that the risk for melanoma include family history, indoor tanning, fair skin, freckles, the number of moles on a your skin, exposure to ultraviolet radiation and severe sunburns. Therefore, one should avoid sunburn and tanning booths.

How about sunscreens? There is a lot of confusion, but here are some facts. Both UVA and UVB cause skin cancer. Therefore, do not use sunscreens that provide protection against UVB only. Get sunscreens that protect for both UVA and UVB.

What is in the sunscreen also matters. Originally, sunscreens contained Zinc Oxide, which does not get absorbed through the skin and therefore, does not have any systemic effects on health. However, this type of sunscreen leaves a thick layer of white material on your skin, which is unaesthetic. Therefore, the pharmaceutical industry came up with new, aesthetically appealing sunscreens.

Unfortunately, these sunscreens typically contain **three** ingredients which get partially absorbed through the skin and are quite harmful: Retinyl palmitate, Oxybenzone, and parabens.

Retinyl palmitate has been shown to increase the rates of cancer. Oxybenzone can cause skin rashes, hives and skin damage. Parabens are linked to an increased risk for breast cancer. Parabens also decrease your testosterone level.

New sunscreen containing micronized Zinc oxide may be a better alternative to traditional Zinc Oxide containing sunscreen for aesthetic reasons.

One should avoid spray sunscreen which causes significant absorption through the lungs and can be quite harmful.

Here are some tips about sunbathing:

- Don't apply any sunscreen while sunbathing. Remember, a sunscreen with SPF of more than 8 will block most UVB and therefore, prevent vitamin D synthesis. In addition, many sunscreens do not block UVA. Therefore, if you apply sunscreen while sunbathing, you may end up with little vitamin D synthesis, and an increased risk of skin cancer.

- Start out sunbathing with about 2-5 minutes on each side, every day.

- Gradually, increase the duration of sun exposure according to your skin tolerance, which depends upon your skin type.

- A good dose of sun exposure is when your skin gets tanned, or slightly reddish, which fades out in about 24 hours. This is also called Minimal Erythema Dose (MED.)

- Be careful not to get a sunburn.

- A good time to sunbath is in the afternoon, between 1-5 PM. Try to avoid the strong sun at noon.

- Sunny days are better than cloudy days for sun-bathing for the following reason: Clouds decrease the intensity of UVB, but not UVA. Therefore, on a cloudy day, you will get mostly UVA and only small amounts of UVB. Remember, UVB is responsible for vitamin D synthesis.

- Glass also interferes with UVB, but not UVA. Therefore, sunbathing indoors, next to glass windows in not a good idea.

- In general, people with dark skin need about 5-6 times the duration of sun exposure as compared to fair-skinned individuals in order to synthesize the same amount of vitamin D.

- The duration of sun exposure can be a bit more during winter months and a little less during summer months.

In addition to sunbathing, try to use sleeve-less shirts and shorts in your every day life, if weather and your culture permits.

Caution:

People with a history of skin cancer should avoid the sun as much as possible and wear sunscreen when they are outdoors.

2. DIET

Diet is *not* a good source of vitamin D. However, you can get some vitamin D from diet. Please note that when you select food, vitamin D should not be the only consideration. You need to take a more comprehensive approach when selecting food, paying attention to overall ingredients.

Different people have different nutritional requirements, depending on numerous factors such as age, genetics, weight, metabolism, physical activity, seasonal variation and medical conditions such as diabetes, cholesterol disorder, high blood pressure, heart disease, Metabolic Syndrome, menopause symptoms, Polycystic Ovary Syndrome, thyroid disorders and other medical conditions.

As I mentioned earlier, modern medicine suffers from "narrow mindedness" in the sense that every expert gives advice according to his/her specialty without looking at the overall person as a whole. That's why there are so many different diets, each conflicting with the other, each claiming to be better than the other.

Consider this scenario: In a magazine article, an expert recommends drinking plenty of orange juice because it contains 100 I.U. of vitamin D per cup. So you start drinking a lot of orange juice without realizing that you're also consuming large quantities of sugar and potassium in the orange juice. If you happen to be diabetic, your glucose values will go through the roof. If you have Metabolic Syndrome and are pre-diabetic, your insulin level will skyrocket. If you're an elderly person with diabetes, high blood pressure and kidney failure, your blood sugar will shoot up and your blood potassium may also become elevated, which if not diagnosed and treated appropriately, can be life threatening. As you can see, you can get in a real mess just because you were myopically focusing on improving your vitamin D level.

So, please beware of all ingredients in a food, not just it's vitamin D content.

With this understanding, let us take a closer look at some foods and their vitamin D contents:

MILK

Natural milk does not contain vitamin D, but milk in the USA and many other countries is fortified with vitamin D.

However, even fortified milk contains only <u>100 I.U. per cup (8 oz or 240 ml).</u> *Drink one to two cups a day.* In this way, you get about 100-200 I.U. of vitamin D and other components of milk in a small to moderate amount. Milk is a good source of calcium. It's also a good source of protein and also contains some natural sugar and some fat.

Milk is a much better choice than soft drinks, which are loaded with sugar or other artificial sweeteners which can have a lot of side-effects. Diet drinks have no real nutritional value. Another disadvantage: soft drinks don't have any vitamin D. People with lactose intolerance obviously should either drink Lactose free milk or avoid milk altogether.

YOGURT

Some yogurts have added vitamin D. Yogurt is also an excellent source of calcium as well as Lactobacillus, a friendly bacteria, which is very important for the health of your intestines.

CHEESE

Some cheeses contain a small amount of vitamin D. Cheeses are fattening and are also loaded with LDL (bad) cholesterol. I advise patients to limit cheeses to reduce weight and also to lower LDL cholesterol.

FISH

Oily fish such as salmon, mackerel and blue fish naturally contain reasonable amounts of vitamin D.
The amount of vitamin D in fish remains unchanged if it is baked, but decreases about 50% if the fish is fried. Also, farm raised salmon has only about 25% of vitamin D as compared to wild salmon.

A word of caution about fish consumption!

Too much fish consumption can lead to mercury poisoning. Fish with high mercury content include shark, whale, swordfish, king mackerel, tilefish and tuna (both fresh and frozen tuna). However, canned tuna doesn't seem to be high in mercury because it consists of smaller, shorter-lived species. Fresh water fish which can be high in mercury include bass, pike, and muskellunge.

Therefore, I recommend caution when consuming fish. Moderation is the key. Avoid those fish that contain high levels of mercury. This is particularly true for pregnant women, lactating women, young children and women of child bearing age, as the developing brain of the fetus and newborn is very susceptible to the injurious effects of mercury.

For this reason, the Food and Drug Administration recommends that pregnant women, breast feeding women and young children should avoid eating fish with high mercury content.

OTHER FOOD ITEMS

Other foods that contain very small amounts of vitamin D include vegetables, meats and egg yolk.

The following food items are supposed to contain the indicated amount of vitamin D

Cod Liver Oil, 1 Tablespoon = 1360, I.U.	Swordfish, cooked, 3 ounces = 566, I.U.	Salmon, cooked (3.5 ounces) = 360, I.U.
Mackerel, cooked (3.5 ounces) = 345, I.U.	Canned Tuna (3.0 ounces) = 200, I.U.	Sardines canned in oil, drained (1.75 ounces) = 250, I.U.
Raw Shiitake Mushrooms (10 ounces) = 76, I.U.	Fortified Milk, one cup (8 ounces or 240 ml) = 100, I.U.	Yogurt, from fortified milk, 6 ounces = 80, I.U.
Margarine, fortified,1 Tablespoon = 60, I.U.	Fortified Orange Juice, one cup (8 ounces or 240 ml) = 100, I.U.	Fortified Cereal 40-80 I.U. per serving.
Egg, 1 whole (vitamin D is found in the yolk) 20, I.U.	Liver of beef, cooked (3.5 ounces) = 15, I.U.	Swiss cheese (1 ounce) = 12, I.U.

I.U. = International Units

3. VITAMIN D SUPPLEMENTS

From a practical perspective, you don't get enough vitamin D from sun exposure and food. As I mentioned earlier, in my clinical practice in Southern California, I have encountered only one young lady who had a good level of vitamin D from sun exposure alone, without any vitamin D supplement. She was a lifeguard at the beach. For the rest of us, vitamin D supplements becomes the major source of vitamin D.

The Starting Dose Of Vitamin D Supplement

The starting dose of vitamin D supplement varies from person to person. It mainly depends on how low your vitamin D level is and how much you weigh. So, please get your vitamin D level checked and then use the following table as a guide to choose the starting dose of vitamin D3.

25 (OH) Vitamin D level in ng/ml	Dose of Vitamin D3
Less than 10	15,000 I.U. a day
10 - 20	12,500 I.U. a day
20 - 30	10,000 I.U. a day
30 - 40	7,500 I.U. a day
41 - 50	5,000 I.U. a day

Your Vitamin D-dose also depends upon your body weight. The heavier you are, the more Vitamin D you need. Why? Because Vitamin D is *fat soluble* and gets trapped in fat. Consequently, less is available for the rest of the body. For this reason, obese people require a larger dose compared to thin people.

The above recommendations are for an average adult, with a weight of about **150 Lbs**. <u>As a guide, add 1000 I.U. for each 20 Lbs. above 150 Lbs. And subtract 1000 I.U. for each 20 lbs. below 150 Lbs.</u>

For some reason, if you cannot get your vitamin D level checked, then here is the formula you can use to calculate the daily dose of vitamin D3. **Use 1000 I.U. for every 20 lbs. of your body weight.**

Pay Attention To The Units On Your Vitamin D Supplement

In the USA, the dose of vitamin D is available in I.U. However, in some parts of the world, vitamin D is available in microgram (mcg).

Here is the conversion factor:

40 I.U. = 1 mcg

For example:

400 I.U. = 10 mcg
1,000 I.U. = 25 mcg.
5,000 I.U. = 125 mcg
10,000 I.U. = 250 mcg
50,000 I.U. = 1,250 mcg or 1.25 mg

Vitamin D2: 50,000 I.U.

When Vitamin D level is below 20, an alternative treatment is to take a high dose of vitamin D2. This is usually given as 50,000 I.U. per week for about 12 weeks.

In the USA, you need a physician's prescription for this dose of vitamin D2. Now vitamin D3 is also available in a dose of 50,000 I.U.

The Maintenance Dose Of Vitamin D Supplement

A common problem arises from traditional medical training which teaches that once your vitamin D stores are replenished, you go back to a daily maintenance dose of 600 I.U. a day. For example, if your vitamin D is very low (let's say less than 15 ng/ml), your physician will likely place you on a high dose of vitamin D2 such as 50,000 I.U. a week for 12 weeks and afterwards, put you back on 600 I.U. a day as a maintenance dose.

Most likely, in the following months, your physician won't check to see what happens to your vitamin D level on this miniscule dose. This kind of practice is based on the medical myth hammered into physicians that once you've replenished vitamin D stores, the problem is somehow cured.

Take a closer look at this myth. Vitamin D stays in your body stores for just a few weeks. Therefore, the "so called cure" of low vitamin D will only last a few weeks and then you'll be back to your usual state of a low level of vitamin D.

For this reason, I check vitamin D level in my patients every three months. What I've discovered is eye opening! In my clinical experience, the maintenance dose of vitamin D depends on the initial starting dose. For example, if a patient requires a high initial starting dose, that patient will need a high maintenance dose. Most people continue to require a high dose of vitamin D to maintain a good level. It makes perfect sense. Why?

It's the overall lifestyle of a person that determines the level of vitamin D. If a person is very low in vitamin D to begin with, it's due to life-style, which in most cases doesn't change after a few weeks of vitamin D therapy. Therefore, it's important to continue a relatively high dose of vitamin D as a maintenance dose, especially in those individuals who are very low in vitamin D to start with.

Most of my patients require a daily dose of 5000 -10,000 I.U. of vitamin D3 to maintain a good level of vitamin D. However, some need up to 15,000 - 20,000 I.U. a day, while others need only 2,000 - 3,000 I.U. a day.

What Type Of Vitamin D?
D3 or D2?

Vitamin D2, also known as ergocalciferol, is of plant origin. On the other hand, Vitamin D3, also known as cholecalciferol, is of animal origin. In the natural state, humans synthesize Vitamin D3 in their skin upon exposure to the sun. Therefore, I recommend Vitamin D3, as this is the physiological type of Vitamin D for humans.

Vitamin D: Oral (Swallowing)
Or
Sublingual (Under The Tongue)

I recommend the SUBLINGUAL (under the tongue) route for absorption of your Vitamin D supplement as compared to oral ingestion (swallowing). Why? Because sublingual absorption takes Vitamin D directly into general circulation, (medically known as systemic circulation), just like when Vitamin D is naturally synthesized in the skin from exposure to the sun.

In contrast, Vitamin D from oral ingestion is absorbed into local circulation (medically known as portal circulation) from the gut, which takes it to the liver first before entering into systemic circulation. In this way, oral ingestion is not very physiological and sublingual absorption is more physiological. This point becomes even more important in people who have problems with digestion, such as people with pancreatitis, Crohn's disease, Irritable Bowel Syndrome, gluten sensitivity, celiac disease and tropical sprue.

It's also a problem for people who take medications that can interfere with intestinal absorption of Vitamin D, such as seizure medicines, cholestyramine, orlistat and also for people with stomach bypass surgery, including those with lap-band procedures.

You can get Sublingual Vitamin D3 from online retailers. One such retailer's address is: http://powerofvitamind.com/sublingual_vitamin_d.html

Monitoring Vitamin D Level

I cannot overemphasize the need for close monitoring of your vitamin D level.

An individual's response to a dose of vitamin D varies widely. As I mentioned before, because vitamin D is fat soluble, it gets trapped in fat. That means there is less vitamin D available for the rest of the body. Therefore, obese people require a larger dose of vitamin D than lean individuals. As vitamin D is fat soluble, it requires normal intestinal mechanisms to absorb fat. If a person has some problem with fat absorption, such as patients with chronic pancreatitis or pancreatic surgery or stomach surgery, then they may not absorb vitamin D adequately.

During summertime, the sun is stronger and many people spend time outdoors. Therefore, the required dose of vitamin D supplement may go down a bit.

In wintertime, the dose of vitamin D may need to go up a bit. However, in a lot of individuals this seasonal variation is little as they mostly stay indoors and apply a good layer of sunscreen when they do go out.

The amount of vitamin D people get from their food also fluctuates considerably. In addition, some people take their vitamin D supplement regularly, while others take it sporadically.

Therefore, I check 25 (OH) vitamin D blood level every 3 months and adjust the dose of vitamin D accordingly. My aim is to achieve and maintain a level of 25 (OH) vitamin D in the range of 50 - 100 ng/ml.

I also check blood calcium to make sure that a person doesn't develop vitamin D toxicity. I recommend monitoring vitamin D and blood calcium level every three months. The blood test for calcium is part of a chemistry panel, usually referred to as CHEM 12 (chemistry 12) or CMP (Comprehensive Metabolic Panel). It's a routine blood test for most people who have an ongoing health issue such as diabetes, hypertension, cholesterol disorder, arthritis, etc.

SPECIAL SITUATIONS

1. STEROIDS

Because steroids lower your vitamin D, I educate my patients to notify me if another doctor places them on a steroid. When someone takes a high dose steroid in an oral form such as Prednisone or in an injectable form such as Solumedrol, Depomedrol or Decadron, I double the dose of vitamin D3 for the duration of steroid intake. In these patients, I check their 25 (OH) vitamin D level every 2 months and change the dose of vitamin D accordingly.

2. CHILDREN AND TEENAGERS

Because human milk doesn't contain any appreciable amounts of vitamin D, infants who are solely breastfed are at high risk for vitamin D deficiency. Therefore, the American Academy of Pediatrics recently raised their recommended daily dose of vitamin D to 400 I.U. in infants who are solely breastfed, beginning at the age of two months.

In most children, a daily dose of vitamin D can be calculated as follows: Use 1000 I.U. of vitamin D3 for every 20 Lbs. of body weight. In addition, it makes sense to use sensible sun exposure, especially in infants and toddlers.

The teenage years are the time when most of your bone growth takes place. Therefore, teenagers need a good dose of vitamin D and calcium. In my opinion, they should be encouraged to spend time outdoors and have sensible sun exposure. In addition, they should also take vitamin D3 according to the formula provided above.

3. PREGNANT AND BREASTFEEDING WOMEN

Pregnant and breast-feeding women are at higher risk for vitamin D deficiency. Low vitamin D in the mother leads to low vitamin D in the infant, with the terrible consequences such as low birth weight, soft skull bones and rickets.

Therefore, for pregnant and breastfeeding women, I check vitamin D level at baseline and monitor it every two months. I treat their low vitamin D as described earlier in this chapter. If blood levels aren't available, then these women should take a dose of at least 5,000 I.U. of vitamin D3 a day.

4. MALABSORPTION SYNDROMES

Low vitamin D is extremely common among people with malabsorption syndromes such as Crohn's disease, Celiac sprue, chronic pancreatitis and intestinal, pancreatic or stomach surgeries.

In these patients, early diagnosis and treatment of vitamin D deficiency is important or they end up developing another disease, called secondary hyperparathyroidism, in which your parathyroid hormone (PTH) gets elevated. PTH is normally secreted by four tiny glands lying low in the neck, behind your thyroid gland. Excess PTH leads to weakening of bones, bone pains and osteoporosis.

In these patients, I check baseline vitamin D level. I find that it is almost always very low. I treat low vitamin D according to my strategy discussed earlier. These patients usually require a *large* dose of vitamin D to meet their vitamin D needs. I strongly recommend Vitamin D3 as *sublingual* preparation in these individuals.

HOW MUCH CALCIUM?

Calcium absorption from the intestines is dependent on vitamin D level. The usual recommended dose of calcium of 1500 mg per day comes from the era when we did not pay any attention to vitamin D and every one was low in vitamin D.

However, things are changing now. If you have a good level of vitamin D, you do not need 1500 mg of calcium every day. In fact, this amount of calcium may be too much for you. That's why sometimes, your blood calcium may become slightly elevated. In that case, you need to lower your calcium intake. Unfortunately, often your physician may tell you to lower the dose of vitamin D.

When you have a good level of vitamin D (more than 50 ng/mL or 125 nmol/L), you need only about 600 - 1000 mg of calcium per day.

Sources Of Calcium

Dairy is the best source of calcium, which includes milk, yogurt and cheese. Each dairy serving has about 300 mg of calcium.
Therefore, all you need is about 3 servings of dairy per day. Other good sources of calcium include bok choy, broccoli, tofu, green snap peas, okra, turnip greens, kale and eggs.

If for some reason you don't consume dairy, such as due to Lactose intolerance, then you need to take calcium supplements. People who suffer from malabsorption syndrome, also need higher doses of calcium supplements.

Among calcium supplements, I recommend calcium citrate, which is cheap and easily available.

VITAMIN D TOXICITY

Every article written in newspapers and magazines about vitamin D always includes an overly scary caution about vitamin D toxicity. The reader gets the impression that it must be a common consequence of vitamin D supplementation. Some readers get so scared, they decide not to take vitamin D supplementation and end up with the health consequences of vitamin D deficiency. What a shame! It's obvious to me that the writers of these magazine and newspaper articles don't actually treat patients with low vitamin D and their knowledge about vitamin D toxicity is very limited and superficial.

What Is Vitamin D Toxicity?

Vitamin D toxicity is defined as "too much vitamin D, causing harm to the body."

What Level Of Vitamin D Causes Damage To The Body?

According to an excellent review article (14) from Queen's University in Kingston, Ontario, Canada, the author concluded that a blood level of 25 (OH) vitamin D more than 300 ng/ml (750 nmol/L) is considered to cause toxicity.
In an animal model (15), blood concentration of vitamin D up to 400 ng/ml (1000 nmol/L) was not associated with any toxicity.

The experts in the field of vitamin D have chosen the normal range of 25 (OH) vitamin D as 30 - 100 ng/ml (75 - 250 nmol/L) to provide a large safety margin.

In an excellent study (16) from the University of Toronto, researchers report 2 cases of high doses of vitamin D.

The first gentleman had been taking 4,000 I.U./day for 3 years followed by 3 years of 8,000 I.U./day. Serum 25 (OH) vitamin D levels averaged 52 ng/ml, while taking 4,000 I.U./day of vitamin D3. While taking 8,000 I.U./day of vitamin D3, mean serum 25 (OH) vitamin D levels were 104 ng/ml. There was *no* evidence of vitamin D toxicity. He maintained a normal level of calcium in the blood and urine over the 6 years of the vitamin D3 intake.

The second gentleman was a 39-year-old man diagnosed with multiple sclerosis. He initiated his own dose-escalation schedule. He increased vitamin D3 dose from 8,000 to 88,000 I.U./day over a period of 4 years. At this extremely high dose, his blood 25 (OH) vitamin D level was 450 ng/ml, and his blood calcium was 2.63 mmol/L (reference range (2.2 - 2.6 mmol/L). As you can see, even at this super-high dose of vitamin D, his serum calcium was only slightly above the upper limit of normal, without any symptoms of toxicity.

At this point, he stopped vitamin D3 supplementation. Two months later, all biochemistry values were within reference ranges; serum 25 (OH) vitamin D concentrations fell by about one-half, to 262 ng/ml. These results help to clarify the human response to higher intakes of vitamin D3.

I have seen several individuals who have been self-administering a daily dose of vitamin D3 as 15,000 to 30,000 I.U. for several years. Their 25 (OH) vitamin D level often gets above 100 ng/ml, but less than 130 ng/ml. None of them have experienced any vitamin D toxicity. Their calcium in the blood remains in the normal range

How Frequent Is Vitamin D Toxicity?

Extremely rare.

In medical literature, cases of vitamin D toxicity are rare.

A case of vitamin D toxicity was reported (17) from All India Institute of Medical Sciences in New Delhi, India. The patient was a 70-year-old woman with a long-standing history of hypertension and diabetes. She presented with decreased appetite, constipation and episodes of transient loss of consciousness. Her total blood calcium was 12.4 mg/dL (normal range 8.5 - 10.5 mg/dL) and vitamin D level was 2016 ng/mL. A retrospective analysis of her treatment history revealed that the patient had received 4 intramuscular injections of 600,000 I.U. each of Architol (vitamin D3), prior to presentation. With treatment, she recovered.

In another excellent study (18) from SheriKashmir Institute of Medical Sciences in Srinagar, India, researchers described 10 cases of vitamin D toxicity over a decade since 2000. The dose of vitamin D ranged from 3.6 million I.U. to 210 million I.U. over periods ranging from 1 - 4 months. These patients presented with vomiting, excessive urination, excessive thirst, confusion and kidney failure. Nine individuals recovered, while one died due to overwhelming infection.

Another study (19) came from Columbia University College of Physicians and Surgeons in New York. Researchers described 9 patients who presented with high blood elevated 25 (OH) vitamin D. All of these individuals reported recently taking an over-the-counter vitamin supplement called Soladek readily available in the Dominican Republic and in Upper Manhattan. Each 5-ml vial of Soladek contains vitamin D_3 (864,000 I.U.) and vitamin A (predominantly retinyl palmitate 123,500 I.U.). Most of these patients had a disorder that can be associated with high calcium level: one had squamous cell cancer of the neck, one had Pneumocystis infection, three had mycobacterial infections, one had lymphoma, one had granulomatous disease and two had hyperthyroidism .
It is pretty obvious that all of these patients with vitamin D toxicity were taking an extremely high dose of vitamin D.

Most of my patients take a daily vitamin D3 dose of 5000 I.U. to 15,000 I.U. (125 mcg to 375 mcg.) I check vitamin D level in all of my patients and have been doing so over the last thirteen years. In the last thirteen years, *I haven't seen a single case of vitamin D toxicity in my patients while they are on vitamin D3 or D2 supplementation!* Most of these patients have a level of 25 (OH) vitamin D less than 100 ng/ml. Rarely, I see someone with a level above 100 ng/ml (250 nmol/L), but less than 130 ng/ml (325 nmol/L.) Even in these patients, blood calcium is almost always normal.

Rarely, I see a patient with a slight increase in calcium level above the normal limit. Simply reducing calcium intake brings the calcium back into the normal range in these patients. I don't consider this slight increase in the calcium level as a case of vitamin D toxicity. My experience is in line with other experts in the field of vitamin D.

Risk Of Toxicity: Over The Counter Vitamin D3 Versus Prescription Vitamin D, Calcitriol (Rocaltrol).

Let me clarify another issue. When medical writers of newspaper and magazine articles talk of vitamin D toxicity, they make a blanket statement about vitamin D supplements, which is a mistake. There are several different preparations of vitamin D supplements. These include Vitamin D3 (cholecalciferol), Vitamin D2 (ergocalciferol), Calcidiol and Calcitriol. Calcitriol is also known as the brand name Rocaltrol.

Calcitriol (Rocaltrol) is a synthetic form of vitamin D and is a drug rather than a supplement. Therefore, it requires a prescription from a physician. It is typically given to patients who have kidney failure and are on dialysis.

Calcitriol (Rocaltrol) is also sometimes prescribed to patients whose parathyroid glands have been removed, often inadvertently by a surgeon during thyroid surgery. Calcitriol (Rocaltrol) is much more potent than natural vitamin D3 or D2 and can sometimes result in vitamin D toxicity. Physicians who prescribe calcitriol (Rocaltrol) are typically aware (and definitely should be aware) of this possibility and monitor their patients for vitamin D toxicity.

Can You Develop Vitamin D Toxicity From Too Much Sun?

The answer is No. You can't develop vitamin D toxicity from too much sun exposure. The reason? Nature is smart. The skin forms as much vitamin D as the body needs. Beyond that, it degrades any excess vitamin D into inactive metabolites. Pretty smart!

How Do You Detect Vitamin D Toxicity?

Vitamin D helps in the absorption of calcium from the intestines. Toxic levels of Vitamin D can cause an increase in blood level of calcium. Thus, vitamin D toxicity manifests itself as a high level of calcium in the blood.

The simplest and the most scientific way to find vitamin D toxicity is to check your calcium and vitamin D level in the blood. Everyone should have his/her vitamin D level and calcium checked every three months.

Symptoms Of Vitamin D Toxicity

Symptoms of vitamin D toxicity are due to increase in the blood level of calcium.

Mild increase in blood calcium level : Usually doesn't cause any symptoms.

Moderate increase in blood calcium : Usually causes non-specific symptoms of nausea, vomiting, constipation, poor appetite, weight loss and weakness. Remember these symptoms can be caused by a variety of other medical conditions as well.

Severe increase in blood calcium level : Causes neurologic symptoms such as somnolence, confusion, even coma and heart rhythm abnormalities, which can be fatal if not treated promptly.

Treatment OF Vitamin D Toxicity

Rarely, I see a patient whose blood calcium goes slightly above the upper limit of normal while on vitamin D supplementation. I lower their calcium intake and repeat a blood test for calcium in a month. In my experience, the reduction in calcium intake brings down calcium into the normal range.

Very rarely, blood calcium remains slightly elevated. I then check parathyroid hormone level. If it is in the normal range, then I further discuss diet with the patient and try to lower calcium intake. Even in these very rare patients, blood calcium normalizes by lowering their calcium intake.

I also keep in mind other causes for elevated blood calcium level such as primary hyperparathyroidism and cancer. I order diagnostic testing in this regard on a case by case basis. If blood calcium is elevated and parathyroid hormone (PTH, intact) is also elevated and both of these values do not normalize with vitamin D supplementation, then that patient is most likely suffering from primary hyperparathyroidism. If parathyroid hormone (PTH, intact) level is normal and the patient continues to have an elevated calcium level, I investigate the possibility of other causes of high calcium such as Cancer, Benign Familial Hypocalciuric Hypercalcemia.

Rarely, high blood calcium may occur due to vitamin D toxicity which can happen if very high doses of vitamin D are used (such as more than 50,000 I.U. per day) for a long period.

Remember, there are many causes of an increase in blood calcium level other than vitamin D toxicity. Two such common causes of high blood calcium are: Primary hyperparathyroidism and cancer. If you have high blood calcium, your physician should thoroughly look into various causes of high blood calcium.

It's important to notify your physician about all the dietary supplements, including vitamin D, which you take. Most physicians don't specifically ask about dietary supplements and often patients don't think to provide this information either. For best medical care, your physician should know all the medicines as well as all the dietary supplements that you take.

If your physician determines that a mild increase in your blood calcium level is due to excessive doses of "over the counter" vitamin D supplementation, as evidenced by a high blood level of 25 (OH) Vitamin D, in consultation with your physician, you should decrease the dose of your calcium intake and vitamin D.
In most cases, simply reducing the calcium intake will bring calcium back into the normal range. If your physician advises you to reduce the dose of vitamin D, you should do so.
Recheck your calcium level in a month or so to make sure that your blood calcium is back to normal. Recheck your vitamin D and calcium in about 3 months to make sure that these levels are good and you haven't swung in the other direction.

If your blood calcium is high due to "prescription vitamin D," such as **calcitriol**, the treatment will depend upon the degree of high blood calcium and your symptoms. Your physician will manage it accordingly. If your calcium level is moderate to severely high, your physician will likely admit you to the hospital for proper treatment of vitamin D toxicity.

References:

1.Yetley EA, Assessing vitamin D status of the U.S. population. *Am J Clin Nutr.* 2008;88(2)558S-564S.

2.Ginde AA, Liu MC, Camargo CA Jr. Demographic differences and trends of vitamin D insufficiency in the US population, 1988-2004. *Arch Intern Med.* 2009;169(6):626- 632.

3.Prentice A. Vitamin D deficiency: a global perspective. *Nutr Rev.* 2008; 66(10 suppl 2): S153-164.

4.Harinarayan CV. *Prevalence* of *vitamin D insufficiency* in postmenopausal south Indian women. *Osteoporos Int.* 2005 Apr;16(4):397-402.

5.Woo J, Lam CW, Leung J, Lau WY, Lau E, Ling X, Xing X, Zhao XH, Skeaff CM, Bacon CJ, Rockell JE, Lambert A, Whiting SJ, Green TJ. Very high rates of vitamin D insufficiency in women of child-bearing age living in Beijing and Hong Kong. *Br J Nutr.* 2008 Jun;99(6):1330-4.

6.Yoshimura N, Muraki S, Oka H, Morita M, Yamada H, Tanaka S, Kawaguchi H, Nakamura K, Akune T. Profiles of vitamin D insufficiency and deficiency in Japanese men and women: association with biological, environmental, and nutritional factors and coexisting disorders: the ROAD study. *Osteoporos Int.* 2013 May 15

7.Al-Mogbel ES. Vitamin D status among Adult Saudi Females visiting Primary Health Care Clinics. *Int J Health Sci (Qassim).* 2012 Jun;6(2):116-26.

8.Martini LA, Verly E Jr, Marchioni DM, Fisberg RM. Prevalence and correlates of calcium and vitamin D status adequacy in adolescents, adults, and elderly from the Health Survey-São Paulo. *Nutrition.* 2013 Jun;29(6):845-50

9.Samuel L, Borrell LN. The effect of body mass index on optimal vitamin D status in U.S. adults: The National Health and Nutrition Examination Survey 2001-2006. *Ann Epidemiol.* 2013 Jul;23(7):409-14

10.Stein EM, Strain G, Sinha N, Ortiz D, Pomp A, Dakin G, McMahon DJ, Bockman R, Silverberg SJ. Vitamin D insufficiency prior to bariatric surgery: risk factors and a pilot treatment study. *Clin Endocrinol (Oxf).* 2009 Aug;71(2):176-83

11.Censani M, Stein EM, Shane E, Oberfield SE, McMahon DJ, Lerner S, Fennoy I. Vitamin D Deficiency Is Prevalent in Morbidly Obese Adolescents Prior to Bariatric Surgery. *SRN Obes.* 2013

12. Bischoff-Ferrari H et al. Current recommended vitamin D may not be optimal. *Am J Clin Nutr*. 2006; 84:18-28.

13. Vieth R, Bischoff-Ferrari H, Boucher BJ, Dawson- Hughes B, Garland CF, Heaney RP, et al. The urgent need to recommend an intake of vitamin D that is effective. *Am J Clin Nutr* 2007; 85:649-50.

14.Jones G. The pharmacokinetics of vitamin D. *Am J Clin Nutr*. 2008 Aug;88(2):582S-586S.

15. Shepard RM, DeLuca HF. Plasma concentrations of vitamin D3 and its metabolites in the rat as influenced by vitamin D3 or 245-hydoxyvitamin D3 intakes. *Arch Biochem Biophys* 1980;202:43-53.

16.Kimball S, Vieth R. Self-prescribed high-dose vitamin D3: effects on biochemical parameters in two men. Ann Clin Biochem. 2008 Jan;45(Pt 1):106-10.

17.Garg G, Khadgwat R, Khandelwal D, Gupta N. Vitamin D toxicity presenting as hypercalcemia and complete heart block: An interesting case report. Indian J Endocrinol Metab. 2012 Dec;16(Suppl 2):S423-5

18.Koul PA, Ahmad SH, Ahmad F, Jan RA, Shah SU, Khan UH. Vitamin d toxicity in adults: a case series from an area with endemic hypovitaminosis d. *Oman Med J*. 2011 May;26(3):201-4

19.Lowe H, Cusano NE, Binkley N, Blaner WS, Bilezikian JP. Vitamin D toxicity due to a commonly available "over the counter" remedy from the Dominican Republic. *J Clin Endocrinol Metab*. 2011 Feb;96(2):291-5

Chapter 14

Vitamin B12 Supplementation

People with Hashimoto's thyroiditis are at risk for Vitamin B12 deficiency due to the following reasons:

In order for Vitamin B12 in food to absorb, we need another substance, called intrinsic Factor (IF), which is synthesized by specialized cells in the stomach, called **parietal cells.** Intrinsic factor (IF) then combines with the ingested Vitamin B12, which is also called the extrinsic factor. The combination of the Intrinsic Factor and the Vitamin B12 (IF-B12) then travels through the intestines, until it reaches the terminal part of the intestine, which is known as the terminal ileum. Here this IF-B12 complex gets absorbed into circulation.

People with Hashimoto's thyroiditis are at increased risk to develop antibodies which **destroy the parietal cells.** These antibodies are called anti-parietal cell antibodies and this condition is called atrophic gastritis. As the parietal cells are destroyed, there is no longer production of Intrinsic Factor (IF). In some individuals, antibodies directly attack IF. Lack of IF leads to impaired absorption of Vitamin B12, which manifests as anemia. This is what we call pernicious anemia.

In addition, patients with Hashimoto's thyroiditis may also have Ulcerative Colitis or Crohn's Disease, which often involves the terminal ileum, the part of the intestine where Vitamin B12 normally gets absorbed. Consequently, there is further impairment with the absorption of Vitamin B12.

Why Is Vitamin B12 Important?

Vitamin B12 is important for the synthesis and regulation of DNA in every cell of the body. In this way, it is important in maintaining the integrity of our genome.

It is particularly important for the health of the brain, nerves, blood cells, gastrointestinal tract, heart and fatty acids metabolism.

What Are The
Symptoms Of Low Vitamin B12?

Low Vitamin B 12 can cause the following symptoms:

1. Lack of energy
2. Tingling and numbness in the feet and hands due to peripheral neuropathy
3. Memory loss
4. Dementia
5. Depression
6. Abnormal gait and lack of balance
7. Anemia
8. Burning of the tongue, poor appetite
9. Constipation alternating with diarrhea, vague abdominal pain
10. Increase in the level of Homocysteine, which is a risk factor for heart disease, stroke, Alzheimer's dementia and bone fractures in the elderly. Low folic acid, low vitamin B6 and genetics are the other contributory factors for raised Homocysteine level.

Who Is At Risk For Low Vitamin B12?

1. Those with gastrointestinal disorders such as atrophic gastritis as I explained above. Also, those with chronic pancreatitis, small intestinal resection or bypass, gluten sensitivity (Celiac disease), Crohn's disease and Ulcerative Colitis.

2. Anyone on a strict vegetarian diet, because vegetables are devoid of Vitamin B12.

3. Anyone on the anti-diabetic drug Metformin (Glucophage).

4. Anyone on stomach medicines such as Prilosec, Prevacid, Protonix, Aciphex, Pepcid, Zantac, Tagamet, etc.

5. Antibiotics can lower Vitamin B12 by interfering with the normal intestinal bacterial flora.

6. Anyone who has undergone stomach surgery.

Vitamin B12 Deficiency Often Remains Undiagnosed

Vitamin B12 deficiency often remains undiagnosed because physicians generally don't think of it as a possibility.

For example, when a diabetic patient complains of tingling in their feet, physicians do all the work-up to diagnose diabetic peripheral neuropathy. They then start you on drug treatment without checking your Vitamin B12 level, even if you are on metformin. In reality, peripheral neuropathy in diabetic patients on metformin is often due to two factors: diabetes itself and Vitamin B12 deficiency.

Vitamin B 12 Deficiency Can Be Diagnosed By A Blood Test

A blood level less than 400 pg/ml indicates Vitamin B12 deficiency. In my clinical experience, patients do much better when their Vitamin B12 level is close to 1000 pg/ml or even above 1000 pg/ml.

What Are Natural Sources Of Vitamin B12?

Animal products are the main natural sources of Vitamin B12. On the other hand, plant-derived food is devoid of Vitamin B12.

Good dietary sources of Vitamin B12 include egg yolk, salmon, crabs, oysters, clams, sardines, liver, brain and kidney. Smaller amounts of Vitamin B12 are also found in beef, lamb, chicken, pork, milk and cheese.

Is There Danger Of Vitamin B12 Overdose?

To my knowledge, there are no reported cases of Vitamin B12 overdose in medical literature. It is a water-soluble vitamin. Any excess amounts gets excreted in the urine.

What Are The Different
Forms Of Vitamin B12 Supplements?

Vitamin B12 supplements are available as oral pills and pills for sublingual (under the tongue) absorption.

I prefer the sublingual absorption route because the absorption of Vitamin B12 from the oral cavity (dissolving in the mouth) is excellent. It bypasses the complicated mechanism of IF-Vitamin B12 complex formation in the stomach, and the healthy terminal ileum, which are required for the *orally* administered vitamin B12.

Vitamin B12 is also available in the form of an injection. You need a prescription from a physician for a Vitamin B12 injection.

Chapter **15**

Managing Hypothyroidism and Hashimoto's Thyroiditis During Pregnancy

When patients with hypothyroidism get pregnant, they need close monitoring and should be under the care of an endocrinologist for the following reasons:

1. The dose of thyroid hormones gets elevated, especially after the first trimester. This is mostly due to weight gain during pregnancy. Therefore, your physician needs to adjust the dose of your thyroid hormones, and monitor your thyroid function closely. I usually see my pregnant hypothyroid patients every two months.

2. During the first trimester, your dose of thyroid hormones may need to go down. This is due to the development of Gestational Hyperthyroidism in some individuals, which is believed to be due to a hormone from the placenta, called HCG (Human Chorionic Gonadotropin), which can mildly stimulate TSH receptors in the thyroid gland and give rise to hyperthyroidism. HCG is also the culprit for morning sickness.

Rarely, Gestational Hyperthyroidism may be due to molar pregnancy, which is an obstetrical condition in which placental tissue grows into a mass in the uterus. A fetus may or may not be present.

3. After delivery, the dose of thyroid hormones usually comes back down to the pre-pregnancy level, as you get rid of the weight gain during pregnancy.

4. During pregnancy, there is an increase in the level of thyroid carrying protein called TBG (thyroid binding globulin).
Therefore, your Total T4 and Total T3 gets elevated, but your Free T4 and Free T3 remain normal and truly reflect your thyroid hormone status. For this reason, be careful if your physician orders Total T4 and Total T3 and starts to label you as having too much thyroid hormone (hyperthyroidism.) During pregnancy, you should insist on having a blood test for Free T4 and Free T3, instead of Total T4 and Total T3.

5. Your physician should also check your blood for TPO (Thyroid Peroxidase) antibodies and TG (Thyroglobulin) antibodies. If elevated, as is the case in patients with Hashimoto's Thyroiditis, you should be monitored closely by a high-risk pregnancy specialist, because these antibodies can cross the placenta and can cause Hashimoto's thyroiditis, hypothyroidism, hyperthyroidism or goiter in the fetus.

6. Women with Hashimoto's Thyroiditis are at increased risk for spontaneous miscarriages.

7. If you had Graves' disease and developed hypothyroidism due to radioactive treatment or surgery, your Graves' disease actually may still be active. Why? Because radioactive treatment or surgery does not treat the underlying autoimmune dysfunction. Therefore, you should have a blood test for TRAB (Thyrotropin Receptor Antibody) during the second half of your pregnancy, which if elevated, puts your fetus at a high risk for developing hyperthyroidism, hypothyroidism or goiter.

8. Stress Management is even more important during pregnancy, because now you have to worry about your baby as well. Please refer to stress management discussed in Chapter 11.

9. Vitamin D supplementation becomes even more important. Why? Because your fetus cannot synthesis its own Vitamin D and is entirely dependent on you for its supply. Therefore, I closely monitor the 25 (OH) Vitamin D level in all of my patients during their pregnancy, following the same principles I discussed earlier in the book.

RECIPES

Recipes

This section contains a number of my original recipes. A doctor talking about recipes. Sounds shocking! I understand your shock.

Let me share my own journey regarding cooking. Until the age of about 35, I did not know much about cooking. Then, my mother came to live with me, as she had become disabled due to a stroke. Back then, there was no Indian restaurant in my town. As a necessity, I started cooking at home, because she did not care for regular American food. As I would cook, my mother would also be in the kitchen in her wheelchair, giving instructions, step by step. The results were pretty good. It encouraged me and I started to *like* cooking.

As an endocrinologist, I realize the important role food plays in our health. I clearly see we are what we eat. Gradually, I got more and more involved in cooking. I did not follow any cook books. I simply followed the basic principles of Indian cooking I learned from my mother and improvised my own recipes.

Now, I love cooking. With the help of my lovely wife, we even grow our own vegetables, herbs and fruits. We also have our own chickens. They are great pets because they lay eggs, keep the yard fertilized, eat snails and children love them.

It is such a pleasure to just walk into the back yard and pick fresh vegetables and herbs. While cooking breakfast, I bath in the morning sun, while doing yoga and meditation. Actually, cooking keeps you in the Now and whenever you are in the Now, you are meditating.

Each and every one of these recipes has been subjected to the taste buds of my wife and some friends. I hope you enjoy them too.

Bon appetite!

BREAKFAST SUGGESTIONS

Yogurt

Put 3-4 tablespoons of Plain, Regular yogurt in a bowl. Add a handful of blueberries, blackberries, raspberries or raisins and walnuts, pecans, shredded almonds or pine nuts. Mix well. You can also add 1-2 tablespoons of honey if you like it sweet.

Feta Cheese

Take 2-3 tablespoons of feta cheese. Add black olives and pine nuts, walnuts or pecans. Optional: You can add mint leaves or basil leaves.

Hard Boiled Eggs

Peel and slice two hard boiled eggs and one Avocado. You can sprinkle salt, black pepper or cayenne pepper, according to your taste.

Tip: You can prepare a few "hard-boiled eggs" ahead and keep them in the refrigerator for a handy, quick snack.

Caution: Use hard-boiled eggs within a few days, definitely within a week or they will spoil.

OMELETS

Basic Omelet

Cooking Time = About 10 minutes

Ingredients:

Eggs = 2
Green onions = 2 (You can use 1/2 of one regular white onion in place of green onions), chopped
Olive oil = 2 tablespoons
Salt = ½ teaspoon

Add olive oil and chopped onions to a medium or large pan. Place it on stove at low heat. Cook for a few minutes until onions have softened and turned yellowish.

Meanwhile, crack open 2 eggs in a bowl. Using a tablespoon, dish out 1 egg yolk and throw it away. Leave one egg yolk. Beat it along with the egg whites. Add the eggs to the pan once onions are done.

Sprinkle the salt. In a few minutes, the eggs start looking like an omelet. With a spatula, turn the omelet over. Don't worry if it breaks down. Just turn the pieces over. Cook for a few minutes and your delicious Omelet is ready.

Mushroom Omelet

Follow the basic omelet recipe, but use a handful of mushrooms after your onions are done. Follow the rest of the recipe.

Spinach Omelet

Follow the basic omelet recipe. Add a handful of washed spinach leaves soon after you pour the beaten eggs in the pan. Cook another couple of minutes. Then fold it, instead of turning it over, so the spinach is all inside. Let it cool off for 2-3 minutes, before you eat.

Bell Pepper Omelet

Follow the basic omelet recipe. Chop 1/2 of a bell pepper (any color) and add when you start with your onions. If you like spicy, you can add ½ teaspoon of Cumin seeds and ¼ to ½ teaspoon of cayenne pepper or black pepper soon after pouring the eggs.

Add a few fresh leaves of cilantro or parsley. Then fold it over, so the chopped bell pepper is all inside. Let it cool off for 2-3 minutes, before you eat.

Avocado Omelet

Peel an avocado and slice it into chunks. Once the basic omelet is ready, add avocado chunks. Add a few fresh leaves of cilantro or parsley. Then fold it over, so the avocado chunks are all inside. Let it cool off for 2-3 minutes, before you eat.
If you like avocados, this will be a morning delight for you. Avocados help to raise your good (HDL) cholesterol and are a good source of protein.

Spicy Omelet

Follow the basic omelet recipe. Right after you add the eggs to the pan, add ¼ to ½ teaspoon of cayenne pepper. Add ½ teaspoon of Cumin seeds. Add a few fresh leaves of cilantro or parsley. You can also use ½ of a jalapeño pepper in place of cayenne pepper.

Scrambled Eggs - Mushrooms

Cooking Time = About 10 minutes

Ingredients:

Eggs = 1-2
Mushrooms = 4, diced
Green onions = 2 or a small regular onion, chopped
Garlic = 1 clove, chopped
Olive oil = 2 tablespoons
Salt = 1/2 teaspoon

Optional:

Fenugreek seeds = 1/2 teaspoon
Cumin seeds = 1/2 teaspoon
Turmeric = 1/2 teaspoon
Clove = 1/4 teaspoon
Cayenne pepper = 1/2 teaspoon OR ½ of a jalapeño, sliced
Mustard, yellow or Dijon = 1/2 teaspoon

In a pan, add olive oil, onions, garlic and salt. Start the stove at low heat and let it cook for about 5 minutes, stirring frequently. Then, add mushrooms and let it cook for another few minutes.

In a bowl, crack open 1 - 2 eggs, beat well and add to the pan. Let cook for a few minutes, stirring frequently. Cool for a couple of minutes before serving.

Optional:

In the beginning, add turmeric, fenugreek seeds, cumin seeds and clove along with the onions. At the end, you can add few cherry tomatoes, fresh cilantro or parsley leaves, fresh mint leaves or fresh basil leaves.

Make it Spicy: In the beginning, add ¼ to ½ teaspoon of cayenne pepper or ½ of a jalapeño pepper in place of cayenne pepper.

Scrambled Eggs - Spinach

Cooking Time = About 10 minutes

Ingredients:

Eggs = 1-2
Spinach = about 1/2 cup
Green onions = 2 or a small regular onion, chopped
Garlic = 1 clove, chopped
Olive oil = 2 tablespoons
Salt = 1/2 teaspoon

Optional:

Cranberries, fresh or dried = a handful
Fenugreek seeds = 1/2 teaspoon
Cumin seeds = 1/2 teaspoon
Turmeric = 1/2 teaspoon
Clove = 1/4 teaspoon
Cayenne pepper = 1/2 teaspoon or ½ of a jalapeño pepper in place of cayenne pepper
Mustard, yellow or Dijon = 1/2 teaspoon

In a pan, add olive oil, onions, garlic and salt. Start the stove at low heat and let it cook for about 5 minutes, stirring frequently. Then add spinach and let it cook for another few minutes. In a bowl, crack open 1 - 2 eggs, beat well and add to the pan. Let cook for a few minutes, stirring frequently. Cool for a couple of minutes before serving.

Optional:

In the beginning, add a few cranberries, turmeric, fenugreek seeds, cumin seeds and clove, along with onions. At the end, you can add cherry tomatoes, fresh cilantro or parsley leaves, fresh mint leaves or fresh basil leaves.

Make it Spicy: In the beginning, add ¼ to ½ teaspoon of cayenne pepper OR ½ of a jalapeño pepper.

Scrambled Eggs - Spinach - Eggplant - Bell Pepper

Cooking Time = About 15 minutes

Ingredients:

Egg = 1-2
Spinach = about 1 cup
Eggplant = 1, preferably Japanese or Chinese, chopped
Bell pepper = 1, any color, preferably red, cut into chunks
Tomatoes = 5 cherry, halved or 1 regular, cut into chunks
Green onions = 2 or a small regular onion, chopped
Garlic = 1 clove, chopped
Mustard, yellow or Dijon = 1 tablespoon
Apple cider vinegar = 1 teaspoon
Olive oil = 2 tablespoons
Salt = 1/2 teaspoon

Optional:

Pine nuts = a handful
Fenugreek seeds = 1/2 teaspoon
Cumin seeds = 1/2 teaspoon
Turmeric = 1/2 teaspoon
Cayenne pepper = 1/2 teaspoon OR ½ of a jalapeño pepper

In a pan, add olive oil, onions, garlic and salt. Start the stove at low heat and add eggplant. Pour mustard and vinegar on eggplant chunks. Cook for about 5 minutes, stirring frequently.

In a bowl, crack open 1 - 2 eggs, beat well and add to the pan. Let cook on low heat for a few minutes, stirring frequently. Once eggs are done, add spinach, tomatoes and bell pepper. Cook for 3-5 minutes on low heat.

<u>Optional:</u>

In the beginning, add turmeric, fenugreek seeds and cumin seeds along with onions. In the end, add pine nuts, fresh cilantro or parsley leaves, fresh mint leaves or fresh basil leaves.

Make it Spicy: In the beginning, add ¼ to ½ teaspoon of cayenne pepper OR ½ of a jalapeño pepper along with onions.

Scrambled Eggs - Bell Pepper - Zucchini

Cooking Time = About 15 minutes

Ingredients:

Eggs = 1-2
Bell pepper = 1/2 diced
Zucchini = 1/2 small, chopped
Tomato = 1, diced
Green onions = 2 or a small regular onion, chopped
Garlic = 1 clove, chopped
Olive oil = 2 tablespoons
Salt = 1/2 teaspoon

Optional:

Fig = 1, ripe
Fenugreek seeds = 1/2 teaspoon
Cumin seeds = 1/2 teaspoon
Turmeric = 1/2 teaspoon
Clove = 1/4 teaspoon
Cayenne pepper = 1/2 teaspoon OR ½ of a jalapeño, sliced
Mustard, yellow or Dijon = 1/2 teaspoon

In a pan add olive oil, zucchini, onions, garlic and salt. Start the stove at low heat and let it cook for about 5 minutes, stirring frequently. Then, add bell pepper and cook for another few minutes.

In a bowl, crack open 1 - 2 eggs, beat well and then add to the pan. Let cook for a few minutes, stirring frequently. Cool for a couple of minutes before serving.

Optional:

In the beginning, add turmeric, fenugreek seeds, cumin seeds, and clove, along with onions. At the end you can add few cherry tomatoes, fresh cilantro or parsley leaves, fresh mint leaves.

Make it Spicy: In the beginning, add ¼ to ½ teaspoon of cayenne pepper OR ½ of a jalapeño pepper and add about 1/2 teaspoon of yellow mustard.

Make it Sweet: At the end, add one ripe fig and fresh basil leaves.

Scrambled Eggs - Bell Pepper - Cauliflower

Cooking Time = About 20 minutes

Ingredients:

Eggs = 1-2
Bell pepper = 1/2 of regular sized bell pepper, any color. Cut into several pieces
Cauliflower = 1/8 of the whole cauliflower head, chopped into 4-6 small pieces
Onion = 1/2 of a medium sized onion, chopped
Garlic = 1 clove, sliced
Olive oil = 3 tablespoons
Vinegar = 1/2 teaspoon
Lemon, fresh = Cut in half
Dijon Mustard (or regular, yellow) = small amount
Salt = 1/2 teaspoon

Optional:

Pine nuts = a handful
Cumin seeds (or powder) or Caraway seeds = 1/2 teaspoon
Turmeric powder = 1/2 teaspoon
Clove powder = 1/4 teaspoon
Black pepper OR Cayenne pepper = 1/2 teaspoon
Cilantro or Basil or Mint leaves = 8 -10

In a regular frying pan, pour 1 cup of water. Add mustard and salt. Squeeze the juice of 1/2 lemon. Stir. Place it on the stove at <u>medium</u> heat. Add cauliflower and cover it. Let it cook for about <u>10</u> minutes. Check only once or twice to make sure the water has not cooked off. Avoid frequent uncovering. It will reduce the amount of steam, which is cooking the cauliflower.

Uncover, lower the heat. Add olive oil, onion, and garlic.

Stir frequently. DO NOT COVER. In about 3-5 minutes, when there is very little water left, add one or two beaten eggs. Scramble it with the spatula. Let it cook for about 3-5 minutes, until eggs are done. Stir frequently.

Add bell pepper and cook for another 3-5 minutes. In the end, add vinegar, a handful of pine nuts and cilantro, basil or mint leaves. Mix well.

Optional: In the beginning, add clove powder, turmeric powder, cumin (or caraway seeds), black pepper OR cayenne pepper.

Scrambled Eggs - Bell Pepper - Green Beans

Cooking Time = About 15 minutes

Ingredients:

Eggs = 1-2
Bell pepper = 1 diced
Green Beans = 10
Tomato = 1, diced
Green onions = 2 or a small, regular onion, chopped
Garlic = 1 clove, chopped
Olive oil = 2 tablespoons
White Vinegar = 1/2 teaspoon

Optional:

Cranberries, fresh or dried = a handful
Fenugreek seeds = 1/2 teaspoon
Cumin seeds = 1/2 teaspoon
Turmeric = 1/2 teaspoon
Cayenne pepper = 1/2 teaspoon OR ½ of a jalapeño

In a pan, add a small amount of water and olive oil. Add green beans, onions and garlic. Start the stove at medium heat and let cook for about 5 minutes, stirring frequently. Do not cover. Then, add tomatoes, bell pepper and white vinegar. Let cook for another few minutes.

In a bowl, crack open 1 - 2 eggs, beat well and add to the pan. Let cook for a few minutes, stirring frequently. Cool for a couple of minutes before serving.

Optional:

In the beginning, add cranberries, turmeric, fenugreek seeds and cumin seeds along with onions. At the end, you can add fresh oregano or thyme leaves.

Make it Spicy: In the beginning, add ¼ to ½ teaspoon of cayenne pepper OR ½ of a jalapeño pepper.

Scrambled Eggs - Green Beans - Eggplant

Cooking Time = About 20 minutes

Ingredients:

Eggs = 1-2
Green beans = 15
Eggplant = 1/2, preferably Japanese or Chinese.
Cinnamon stick = 1
Tomato = 1, medium size
Yogurt = Plain, 2-3 tablespoons
Garlic = 1 clove, sliced
Olive oil = 3 tablespoons
Lemon, fresh = Cut into two halves
Dijon Mustard (or regular, yellow) = small amount
Salt = 1/2 teaspoon

Optional:

Pine nuts = a handful
Bay leaf = 1
Cumin seeds (or powder) or Caraway seeds = 1/2 teaspoon
Turmeric powder = 1/2 teaspoon
Cloves powder = 1/4 teaspoon
Black pepper OR Cayenne pepper = 1/2 teaspoon
Cilantro or Basil or Mint leaves = 8-10

In a regular frying pan, pour 1/2 cup of water. Add mustard and salt. Squeeze 1/2 lemon. Stir and cook at <u>medium</u> heat. Add green beans, eggplant, cinnamon stick and bay leaf. DO NOT COVER. Let cook for about <u>5</u> minutes. Stir occasionally. Lower the heat. Add olive oil, garlic, yogurt and tomato.

Stir frequently. DO NOT COVER. In about <u>10</u> minutes, add one or two beaten eggs. Scramble it with a spatula. Let it cook for another 3 - 5 minutes, until eggs are done. Stir frequently. In the end, add a handful of pine nuts and cilantro leaves (or basil or mint leaves).

<u>Optional</u>:

In the beginning, add bay leaf, clove powder, turmeric powder, cumin (or caraway seeds), powdered black pepper (or powdered cayenne pepper).

Scrambled Eggs - Bell Pepper - Zucchini - Daikon Radish

Cooking Time = About 15 minutes

Ingredients:

Eggs = 1-2
Bell pepper = 1/2, diced
Zucchini = 1/2, sliced
Daikon Radish = 4 inch piece, peeled and cut in small pieces
Green onions = 2 or a small regular onion, chopped
Garlic = 1 clove, chopped
Olive oil = 2 tablespoons
Salt = 1/2 teaspoon

Optional:

Pine nuts = a handful
Fenugreek seeds = 1/2 teaspoon
Cumin seeds = 1/2 teaspoon
Turmeric = 1/2 teaspoon
Clove = 1/4 teaspoon
Cayenne pepper = 1/2 teaspoon OR ½ of a jalapeño, sliced
Mustard, yellow or Dijon = 1/2 teaspoon
Cherry tomatoes = 5-8
Fresh cilantro, mint or basil leaves = 8-10
Figs = 2 ripe

In a frying pan, add olive oil, zucchini, Daikon radish and onions. Place the pan on stove at low heat.

Optional: Add garlic, turmeric, fenugreek seeds, cumin seeds, and clove.

Sprinkle salt. Let cook for about 5 minutes, stirring frequently. Then, add bell pepper and let cook for another few minutes.

In a bowl, beat 1 - 2 eggs and then add to the pan. Let it cook for a few minutes, stirring frequently. Let it cool for a couple of minutes before serving.

Optional:

At the end, add a few cherry tomatoes, pine nuts, fresh cilantro, mint or basil leaves.

Make it Spicy: In the beginning, add cayenne pepper OR jalapeño pepper and add mustard.

Make it Sweet: Add two ripe figs, chopped and a few fresh basil leaves.

Scrambled Eggs - Pumpkin

Cooking Time = About 15 minutes

Ingredients:

Eggs = 1 - 2
Pumpkin, fresh = 10 small slices, about 1/4 inch thick, 2 inches wide and 2 inches long, peeled.
Celery Stick = 1, cut into small pieces
Olive oil = 2 tablespoons
Vinegar = 1/2 teaspoon
Lemon, fresh = Cut in half
Mustard, regular, yellow = small amount
Salt = 1 teaspoon
Cumin seeds (or powder) or Caraway seeds = 1 teaspoon
Garlic = 1 clove, sliced

Optional:

Black Pepper OR Cayenne pepper = 1/2 teaspoon.

A wok works better, but you can use a regular frying pan. Add olive oil, pumpkin and celery slices to the wok. Place it on the stove at medium heat. Stir frequently. DO NOT COVER. In about 10 minutes, pumpkin slices will be done: softened but not mushy.

Turn the heat down to low. Add the mustard and squeeze the juice of 1/2 lemon directly on the pumpkin slices. Add vinegar, garlic, cumin seeds, and salt. Let it cook another 2-3 minutes, stirring frequently.

Add beaten eggs to the wok. After a minute, scramble it. Cook for another 2 - 3 minutes.

Optional:

Make it Hot: In the beginning, add Cayenne OR Black Pepper on the pumpkin slices.

Scrambled Eggs - Mushroom - Okra - Daliya

Cooking Time = About 20 minutes

Ingredients:

Eggs = 1-2
Mushrooms, Shiitake = 2, each cut into large pieces.
Okra = 8-10, each sliced into 2-3 pieces, like you slice a cucumber.
Daliya split = 2 tablespoons. (Daliya is roasted chickpeas you can get from an India/Pakistani grocery store.)
Onion = 1/2 of a medium sized onion, chopped
Garlic = 1 clove, sliced
Olive oil = 3 tablespoons
Olives = Black, pitted; 6-8, cut into small pieces.
Vinegar, Balsamic = 1/2 teaspoon
Lemon, fresh = Cut in half
Salt = 1/2 teaspoon
Cumin seeds (or powder) or Caraway seeds = 1/2 teaspoon
Turmeric powder = 1/2 teaspoon
Basil leaves = 8 -10 fresh or 1 tablespoon of dried leaves

Optional:
Black pepper OR Cayenne pepper = 1/2 teaspoon
Clove powder = 1/4 teaspoon

In a regular frying pan, add two tablespoons of olive oil, onion, and garlic. Cook at low heat until onions turn yellowish and soft, which takes about 5 minutes.

In frying pan, add 1 cup of water. Add cumin seeds, turmeric, and salt. Squeeze the juice of 1/2 lemon.

Add okra and daliya. Stir and cover. Let it cook for about <u>10</u> minutes on low heat. Check only once or twice to make sure the water has not cooked off. Avoid frequent uncovering. It will reduce the amount of steam, which is cooking the okra and daliya.

Add one or two beaten eggs. Scramble it with a spatula. Let it cook for about 3-5 minutes, until eggs are done. Stir frequently.

Add mushrooms, olives and basil leaves. Add one tablespoon of olive oil and 1/2 teaspoon of Balsamic vinegar. Mix well. Cook for another 1-2 minutes.

<u>Optional</u>: In the beginning, add clove powder, black pepper OR cayenne pepper.

Scrambled Eggs - Bell Pepper - Green Beans

Cooking Time = About 15 minutes

Ingredients:

Eggs = 1-2
Bell pepper = 1 diced
Green Beans = 10
Tomato = 1, diced
Green onions = 2 or a small, regular onion, chopped
Garlic = 1 clove, chopped
Olive oil = 2 tablespoons
White Vinegar = 1/2 teaspoon

Optional:

Cranberries, fresh or dried = a handful
Fenugreek seeds = 1/2 teaspoon
Cumin seeds = 1/2 teaspoon
Turmeric = 1/2 teaspoon
Cayenne pepper = 1/2 teaspoon OR ½ of a sliced jalapeño

In a pan, add a small amount of water and olive oil. Add green beans, onions and garlic. Start the stove at medium heat and let cook for about 5 minutes, stirring frequently. Do not cover. Then, add tomatoes, bell pepper and white vinegar. Let cook for another few minutes.

In a bowl, crack open 1 - 2 eggs, beat well and add to the pan. Let cook for a few minutes, stirring frequently. Cool for a couple of minutes before serving.

Optional:
In the beginning, add cranberries, turmeric, fenugreek seeds and cumin seeds along with onions. At the end, you can add fresh oregano or thyme leaves.
Make it Spicy: In the beginning, add ¼ to ½ teaspoon of cayenne pepper OR ½ of a sliced jalapeño pepper.

Scrambled Eggs - Broccoli - Eggplant

Cooking Time = About 15 minutes

Ingredients:

Egg = 1-2
Broccoli = about 1 cup
Eggplant = 1, preferably Japanese or Chinese, chopped
Onion = a small regular onion, chopped
Garlic = 1 clove, chopped
Olive oil = 2 tablespoons

Optional:

Pine nuts = a handful
Fenugreek seeds = 1/2 teaspoon
Cumin seeds = 1/2 teaspoon
Turmeric = 1/2 teaspoon
Cayenne pepper = 1/2 teaspoon OR ½ of a jalapeño pepper
Fresh cilantro or parsley leaves,
Fresh mint leaves or fresh basil leaves.
Cayenne pepper = 1/2 teaspoon OR ½ of a sliced jalapeño

In a pan, add one cup of water. Start the stove at low heat and add broccoli, eggplant, onions and garlic. Cover and cook for about 5 minutes.

In a bowl, crack open 1 - 2 eggs, beat well and add to the pan. Let cook on low heat for a few minutes, stirring frequently. Once eggs are done, add olive oil. Cook for 1-2 minutes on low heat.

Optional:
In the beginning, add turmeric, fenugreek seeds and cumin seeds along with onions. In the end, add pine nuts, fresh cilantro or parsley leaves, fresh mint leaves or fresh basil leaves.
Make it Spicy: In the beginning, add ¼ to ½ teaspoon of cayenne pepper OR ½ of a sliced jalapeño pepper along with onions.

Scrambled Eggs - Green Beans - Bell Pepper - Tomatoes - Turnip

Cooking Time = About 15 minutes

Ingredients:

Eggs = 1-2
Green beans = 4-6
Bell pepper = 1/2, diced
Tomatoes = 1-2, diced
Turnip = 1/2, peeled and diced
Green onions = 2 or a small regular onion, chopped
Garlic = 1 clove, chopped
Olive oil = 2 tablespoons
Salt = 1/2 teaspoon
Lemon = Cut in half.

Optional:

Fenugreek seeds = 1/2 teaspoon
Cumin seeds = 1/2 teaspoon
Turmeric = 1/2 teaspoon
Cayenne pepper = 1/2 teaspoon OR ½ of a jalapeño, sliced
Mustard, yellow or Dijon = 1/2 teaspoon
Fresh cilantro leaves = 8-10

In a frying pan, add olive oil, 1/2 cup of water, turnip, onion, garlic, and salt. Squeeze lemon directly onto the pan.

Optional: Add fenugreek seeds, cumin seeds, turmeric, cayenne pepper and mustard.

Cover and cook on low heat for about 10 minutes, stirring occasionally to make sure water is still there. Then, add bell pepper, green beans, and tomatoes. Let it cook for another few minutes, uncovered. Add beaten eggs to the pan. After a minute, scramble it Cook for another 2 - 3 minutes. In the end, add cilantro leaves.

LUNCH OR DINNER

You can use any of the scrambled eggs recipes for lunch or dinner.

Lettuce Wraps: Cheese - Avocado - Eggs - Mango

Ingredients:

Lettuce = 1 head of Iceberg lettuce
Cheese, feta or cottage = a small amount
Avocado = 1, peeled, sliced
Eggs= 2, boiled, peeled, sliced (egg whites only)
Mango (preferably <u>Kent</u> variety from Mexico, available at Indian grocery stores during summer) = 1 ripe, peeled, cut into slices
Salt = a tiny amount

      Gently peel off a leaf from the lettuce head. Place the mango slices, cheese, avocado slices and egg slices in the center of the lettuce leaf. Sprinkle a tiny amount of salt. Roll up the lettuce leaf into a wrap. You can make about 4 wraps with this recipe.

SALADS

Salad 1 (Cucumber - Tomato - Yogurt Salad)

Ingredients:

Yogurt, plain = 4 tablespoons
Tomatoes, cherry = 6 - 10
Cucumber = 1 medium sized, cut into pieces
Green Onion = 1 sliced. Also use green portion
Salt = 1/2 teaspoon
Cumin seeds = 1/2 teaspoon
Mint leaves or basil leaves (preferably fresh) = a few

Add yogurt to a medium sized bowl. Dilute it by adding and mixing 2 tablespoons of water. Then, add onion, cucumber, cumin seeds, salt and mix well. Then mix in tomatoes and mint leaves. Your salad is ready.

Salad 2 (Cucumber - Tomato - Avocado Salad)

Ingredients:
Lettuce = a few leaves, chopped
Cucumber = 1/2, sliced
Tomato = 1 medium, cut into large pieces OR about 10 cherry tomatoes, whole
Avocado = 1, peeled, sliced
Onion = regular, 1/2, peeled, cut into slices
Mint leaves or Cilantro leaves = a few, preferably fresh
Balsamic Vinegar = a tiny amount
Lime or Lemon = 1, cut in half
Salt = a tiny amount

In a medium size bowl, add chopped lettuce. Then, add chopped onion, tomatoes and avocado. Mix well. Add mint or cilantro leaves. Sprinkle salt and a tiny amount of Balsamic Vinegar. In the end, squeeze lime. Mix well.

Salad 3 (Olive - Pine Nut - Avocado Salad)

Ingredients:

Olives, black or green = 8-10
Pine nuts = a handful
Avocado = 1, peeled, sliced
Lettuce = a few leaves, chopped
Tomato = 1 medium, cut into large pieces OR about 10 cherry tomatoes, whole
Balsamic Vinegar = a tiny amount
Lime or Lemon = 1, cut in half
Salt = a tiny amount.

In a bowl, add chopped lettuce. Squeeze lemon juice and sprinkle salt and a tiny amount of Balsamic Vinegar. Then add pine nuts, olives, tomatoes and avocado. Mix well.

Salad 4 (Papaya - Spinach - Pine Nut Salad)

Ingredients:

Lettuce, Romaine = half cup, chopped
Arugula = half cup, chopped
Spinach, baby = half cup
Cucumber = 1/2, sliced
Papaya = 1, small, peeled, seeds removed and cut into chunks
Tomato = 1, medium, cut into large pieces OR about 10 cherry tomatoes, whole
Pine nuts = a handful
Balsamic Vinegar = a tiny amount
Lime or Lemon = 1, cut in half

In a bowl, add baby spinach, chopped lettuce and arugula. Squeeze lemon juice and add a tiny amount of Balsamic Vinegar. Then add cucumber, pine nuts and tomatoes. In the end, add papaya. Mix gently.

Healthy Crepes

Cooking Time = About 3 - 5 minutes for one crepe

Recipe makes 4 Crepes.

Ingredients:

Moong Daal Flour = 2 tablespoons
Besan = 2 tablespoons
Almond flour = 2 tablespoons
Egg = 1
Hiamalayan Salt or Sea Salt = 1/2 teaspoon

You can get Moong Daal and Besan from an Indian/Pakistani Grocery store.

Optional:
Cumin seeds (or powder) or Caraway seeds = 1/2 teaspoon
Black pepper Or Cayenne pepper.= 1/2 teaspoon
Garlic = 1 clove, thinly sliced.

In a bowl, pour Moong daal flour, Besan and Almond flour, add small amount of water (about 1/2 cup), mix well. Then break one egg into the bowl. Mix well. You may need to add a little more water, till the consistency of the batter is runny.

Put a skillet on low heat. Wait a few minutes until the skillet is mildly hot. Pour about 1/4 of the batter on the skillet. Move skillet from side to side, so the batter spreads out evenly. Let it cook until it looks all dried up and edges have turned brownish and rolled-up. It takes a few minutes. With a pancake spatula, turn it over. Let it cook for another couple of minutes.

Remove crepe from skillet into a plate. Let it cool of for a minute or so. then roll it up. You can also add a filling before you roll up.

<u>Optional</u>:
In the beginning, add cumin (or caraway seeds), black pepper OR cayenne pepper and garlic in the bowl.
Fillings for Crepes

Here are some ideas about fillings:
1. Cut an avocado into small pieces. Add black pepper, salt, and cayenne pepper (as optional). Add a few Cilantro leaves. Squeeze a lime or lemon.
2. A handful of nuts such as cashews, walnuts, sliced almonds, pine-nuts, and dried fruits such as cranberries, cherries, apricots or shredded coconut.
3. Cheese
4. Salad
5. Left-over yellow chicken pieces
6. Ground beef/ground turkey

See recipes for yellow chicken and ground beef/turkey, later in the book.

Pumpkin Z-Fries

Cooking Time = About 15 minutes

Ingredients:

Pumpkin, fresh = Cut into the size of French Fries, about 20 - 25,
some peeled and some unpeeled
Olive oil = 2 tablespoons
Cheddar cheese, shredded = a handful
Mustard, Dijon = 3 teaspoons
Vinegar = 1/2 teaspoon

Optional:

Garlic powder = 1 teaspoon
Salt = 1/2 teaspoon
Cumin seeds (or powder) or Caraway seeds = 1 teaspoon
Black Pepper = 1 teaspoon OR Cayenne pepper = 1/2 teaspoon

Place a frying pan on medium heat. Warm olive oil and
then, add pumpkin fries. Add Dijon mustard directly on the
pumpkin fries.

Optional: Add vinegar, garlic, cumin seeds, salt and black OR
cayenne pepper.

Cook for about 10 minutes. DO NOT COVER. Turn the
pumpkin fries over a few times, so they don't get burned.

Turn the heat down to low. Sprinkle a handful of shredded
cheddar cheese. It will melt in a couple of minutes. Place Pumpkin
Z-Fries on paper towel to soak up excess oil.

Pumpkin Z-Fries - Scrambled Eggs - Eggplant

Cooking Time = About 15 minutes

Ingredients:

Eggs = 2
Pumpkin, fresh = Cut into the size of French Fries, about 20 - 25, some peeled and some unpeeled
Eggplant = 1 Japanese or Chinese or 2 small round ones; sliced
Olive oil = 3 tablespoons
Cheddar cheese, shredded = a handful
Mustard, Dijon = 3 teaspoons
Vinegar = 1/2 teaspoon

Optional:
Garlic powder = 1 teaspoon
Salt = 1/2 teaspoon
Cumin seeds (or powder) or Caraway seeds = 1 teaspoon
Onion, Green = 2, chopped. (You can use a small regular onion instead)
Black Pepper = 1 teaspoon OR Cayenne pepper = 1/2 teaspoon
Fresh or dried thyme, oregano, mint OR basil leaves

In a pan, add olive oil, pumpkin fries, and eggplant slices. Add mustard directly on the pumpkin fries.

Optional: Add vinegar, garlic, cumin seeds, salt and black or cayenne pepper.

Cook for about 10 minutes on medium heat. DO NOT COVER. Turn the pumpkin fries and eggplant slices over a few times, so they don't get burned. Then, turn the heat down to low. Sprinkle in a handful of shredded cheddar cheese. In a few minutes, add onions and beaten eggs to the pan. Let it cook about 1 minute, then scramble the eggs with a spatula. Cook for another 2 - 3 minutes, stirring frequently. In the end, add fresh or dried oregano, thyme, mint or basil leaves.

Zucchini Z-Fries - Avocado

Cooking Time = About 15 minutes

Ingredients:

Zucchini, fresh = Unpeeled, cut into the size of French Fries, about 20-25
Avocado = 1, peeled, sliced
Cherry tomatoes = about 10
Olive oil = 3 tablespoons
Cheddar cheese, shredded = a handful
Mustard, Dijon = 4-5 teaspoons
Garlic powder = 1 teaspoon
Onion, Green = 2, chopped (You can use a small regular onion instead.)

Optional:

Salt = 1/2 teaspoon
Clove powder = 1/2 teaspoon
Cumin seeds (or powder) or Caraway seeds = 1 teaspoon
Black Pepper = 1 teaspoon OR Cayenne pepper = 1/2 teaspoon
Cilantro leaves = 8-10 fresh or dried = 1 teaspoon

In a regular frying pan, add olive oil and zucchini fries . Sprinkle garlic powder and add mustard directly on the zucchini fries.

Optional : Add clove powder, cumin seeds, salt and black or cayenne pepper directly on the zucchini fries.

Cook for about 5 minutes on medium heat. DO NOT COVER. Turn the zucchini fries over a few times, so they don't get burned. Sprinkle a handful of shredded cheddar cheese directly on the zucchini fries. Once the cheese melts, remove the zucchini fries onto a plate. Top it with chopped onions, cherry tomatoes, avocado slices and cilantro leaves.

Pumpkin Stir Fry

Cooking Time = About 15 minutes

Ingredients:

Pumpkin, fresh = 10 small slices, about 1/4 inch thick, 2 inches wide and 2 inches long, peeled
Celery Stick = 1, cut into small pieces
Olive oil = 2 tablespoons
Vinegar = 1/2 teaspoon
Lemon, fresh = Cut in half.
Mustard, regular, yellow = small amount
Salt = 1 teaspoon
Cumin seeds (or powder) or Caraway seeds = 1 teaspoon
Garlic = 1 clove, sliced
Black Pepper = 1 teaspoon OR Cayenne pepper = 1/2 teaspoon

Optional:
Avocado slices
Mint or Basil leaves = 8-10

A wok works better, but you can use a regular frying pan. Warm olive oil on medium heat. Add pumpkin slices and celery slices. Stir frequently. DO NOT COVER. In about 10 minutes, pumpkin slices will be done: softened but not mushy.

Turn the heat down to low. Add mustard and 1/2 lemon juice directly on the pumpkin slices. Add vinegar, garlic, cumin seeds, salt and cayenne pepper (or black pepper) to the wok. Let it cook another 2-3 minutes, stirring frequently.

Optional:
For variety, add Avocado slices at the end. Let it cook another 2-3 minutes, stirring frequently. In the end, add a few Mint or Basil leaves.

Cauliflower - Pumpkin - Turnip Stir Fry

Cooking Time = About 15 minutes

Ingredients:

Pumpkin, fresh = 15 small slices, about 1/4 inch thick, 2 inches wide and 2 inches long, peeled
Cauliflower = 3 - 5 florets
Turnip = 1/2, peeled and cut into small slices
Celery Stick = 1, cut into small slices
Olive oil = 2 tablespoons
Vinegar = 1/2 teaspoon
Lemon, fresh = Cut in half
Mustard, regular, yellow = small amount
Salt = 1 teaspoon
Cumin seeds (or powder) or Caraway seeds = 1 teaspoon
Garlic = 1 clove, sliced
Mint leaves Or Basil leaves, fresh = 8-10 OR dried = 1 teaspoon

Optional
Black Pepper = 1 teaspoon OR Cayenne pepper = 1/2 teaspoon

A wok works better, but you can use a regular frying pan instead. Place the wok on <u>medium</u> heat. Add olive oil, pumpkin slices, turnip slices, cauliflower florets and celery slices to the wok. Stir frequently. DO NOT COVER. In about 10 minutes, pumpkin slices will be done: softened but not mushy.

Turn the heat down to low. Add mustard and 1/2 lemon juice directly on the pumpkin slices. Add vinegar, garlic, cumin seeds and salt.

Optional: Add cayenne pepper OR black pepper to the wok.

Let it cook another 2-3 minutes, stirring frequently.

Zucchini - Eggplant - Avocado Delight

Cooking Time = About 15 minutes

Ingredients:

Zucchini = 1 medium size, unpeeled, sliced
Eggplant = 1 small, preferably Japanese or Chinese, sliced
Avocado = 1, peeled, sliced into chunks
Yogurt = Plain, 2 tablespoons
Tomato = 1 medium size, sliced
Onion = 1/2 of a medium sized onion
Olive oil = 3 tablespoons

Optional:

Walnuts or pecans = a handful
Clove, powder = a pinch
Garlic = 1 clove, sliced
Cumin seeds (or powder) or Caraway seeds = 1/2 teaspoon
Turmeric powder = 1/2 teaspoon
Black pepper OR Cayenne pepper = 1/2 teaspoon
Oregano, thyme or rosemary leaves = about 1 teaspoon

In a regular frying pan on <u>medium</u> heat, add olive oil and chopped onions. Stir frequently. In about 3-5 minutes, onion will turn yellowish.

Lower the heat. Add sliced Zucchini and eggplant. After about 2-3 minutes, add yogurt. Let it cook for about 10 minutes on low heat. DO NOT COVER. Stir frequently.

Add Avocado slices and tomato slices. Cook for another couple of minutes. In the end, add walnuts and oregano or thyme or rosemary leaves.

Optional: In the beginning, add clove powder, turmeric powder, cumin (or caraway seeds), black pepper, cayenne pepper.

Eggplant - Bell Pepper - Daikon Radish

Cooking Time = About 15 minutes

Ingredients:

Eggplant = 1 small, preferably Japanese or Chinese, sliced
Bell pepper = 1/2, cut into pieces
Daikon radish = about a 4 inch piece, peeled and cut into pieces
Yogurt = Plain, 2 tablespoons
Tomato = 1 medium size, sliced
Olive oil = 3 tablespoons
Mustard - yellow or Dijon = a small amount

Optional:

Cumin seeds (or powder) or Caraway seeds = 1/2 teaspoon
Turmeric powder = 1/2 teaspoon
Black pepper OR Cayenne pepper = 1/2 teaspoon
Basil or thyme leaves = 8-10

In a regular frying pan, add 1/2 cup of water, olive oil, eggplant and Daikon radish. Put on low heat, cover and stir only a couple of times. In about 5 minutes, uncover and add yogurt and tomato.

Optional: Add cumin (or caraway seeds), black pepper OR cayenne pepper.

Cook for about 5 minutes on low heat. DO NOT COVER. Stir frequently.

Add bell pepper and cook for about 2-3 minutes. Add a small amount of mustard and cook for another 2-3 minutes. In the end, add basil leaves or thyme leaves.

Zucchini - Bell Pepper - Green Beans - Mushroom

Cooking Time = About 15 minutes

Ingredients:

Zucchini = 1, small, unpeeled, sliced
Bell pepper, red = 1, cut into pieces
Green beans = small, 8-10
Mushrooms = white, 5, cut into halves
Tomato = 1 medium, sliced
Onion = 1 small, chopped
Olive oil = 1 tablespoon
Mustard - yellow or Dijon = a small amount
Vinegar, Balsamic = a small amount

Optional:

Cumin seeds (or powder) or Caraway seeds = 1/2 teaspoon.
Turmeric powder = 1/2 teaspoon.
Black pepper OR Cayenne pepper = 1/2 teaspoon.
Basil or Oregano leaves = 8-10

In a regular frying pan, add 1/2 cup of water, olive oil, onion and mustard. Put on low heat, cover and stir only a couple of times. In about 5 minutes, uncover and add green beans, zucchini and tomatoes. Cook for about 5 minutes on medium heat. DO NOT COVER. Stir frequently.

Then, add bell pepper and mushrooms. Cook for about 2-3 minutes. In the end, add basil leaves or thyme leave and sprinkle with a small amount of vinegar.

Optional:
In the beginning, add cumin (or caraway seeds), black pepper OR cayenne pepper.

Cauliflower, Bell Pepper, Green Beans, Cherry Tomatoes and Green Grapes

Cooking Time = About 15 minutes

Ingredients:

Cauliflower = 1/8 of the whole cauliflower head, chopped into 4-6 small pieces
Bell pepper = 1/2 of regular sized bell pepper, any color. Cut into 4-5 chunks
Eggplant = 1/2 of a Chinese or Japanese eggplant, cut into chunks
Green grapes = about 20
Green Beans, small = 5-10
Cherry Tomatoes = 5-10
Onion = 1/2 of a regular sized onion
Garlic = 1 clove, sliced
Olive oil = 3 tablespoons
Mustard, Dijon, (or regular, yellow) = small amount
Salt = 1/2 teaspoon
Pine nuts = a handful
Cilantro or basil = 1/2 teaspoon

Optional:
Cumin seeds (or powder) or Caraway seeds = 1/2 teaspoon
Turmeric powder = 1/2 teaspoon
Black pepper OR Cayenne pepper = 1/2 teaspoon.

In a regular frying pan on low heat, add olive oil and 1/2 cup of water. Add mustard, salt, cauliflower and eggplant, and cover. Let it cook for about 10 minutes. Check only once or twice to make sure water is still in there. Uncover and raise the heat to medium. Add onion, garlic, cherry tomatoes, green beans and grapes. Stir frequently. DO NOT COVER. Add a handful of pine nuts, and basil OR cilantro leaves.

Optional: In the beginning, add cumin (or caraway seeds), turmeric, black pepper OR cayenne pepper.

5 - Leaf Saag

Cooking time = about 60 minutes

Ingredients:

Spinach, baby = 4 cups, chopped
Mustard greens = 6 cups, chopped
Daikon Radish Leaves = 3 cups, chopped
Arugula = 1 cup, chopped
Turnip Leaves = 1 cup, chopped
Daikon Radish = 1, peeled, chopped
Olive oil = 10 tablespoons
Butter = 1 stick
Onion = 2 medium, chopped
Garlic = 2 cloves, sliced
Vinegar = Any type, preferably Balsamic, 1 teaspoon
Salt = 1 teaspoon
Turmeric powder = 1/2 teaspoon
Cilantro leaves = a few
Lime or lemon = 1, cut in half

Optional:

Cumin seeds = 1 teaspoon
Clove powder = 1/2 teaspoon
Black pepper= 2 teaspoons OR Cayenne pepper = 1 teaspoon

    In a large pot, add olive oil. Then add two chopped onions, garlic and salt. Cook on low heat for about 5 minutes, stirring frequently, until the onions have turned yellowish brown.

    Add spinach, mustard greens, Daikon radish and Daikon radish leaves, turnip leaves, arugula, turmeric powder, salt and vinegar.

    Cook for about 45 minutes at low heat, uncovered, stirring frequently until it is not runny and has thick consistency.

Then, pour it into a blender and grind on low until all leaves are well ground. Pour it back into the large pot.

Add 1 stick of butter. Cook for another 15 - 20 minutes on low heat, uncovered, until you start to see oil separating at the periphery.

In the end, add cilantro. Squeeze and add lime or lemon. Mix well. Let it sit for about 15 minutes before serving.

Optional:
In the beginning, add black pepper OR cayenne pepper and clove powder and cumin seeds.

Mixed Lentils

Cooking time = about 60 minutes

Ingredients:

Lentils Urud (preferably whole, with scales) = 1 cup
Lentils Moong (preferably whole, with scales) = 1 cup
(You may need to go to an Indian-Pakistani grocery store to get
these special variety of lentils or try the internet)
Spinach, baby = 4 cups, chopped
Celery = 1 stalk, chopped.
Olive oil = 10 tablespoons
Onion = 1 medium, chopped
Garlic = 2 cloves, sliced
Cinnamon = 1 stick
Vinegar = Any type, preferably Balsamic, 1 teaspoon
Salt = 1 teaspoon
Turmeric powder = 1/2 teaspoon
Fenugreek (or Methi) seeds = 1/2 teaspoon
Cilantro or oregano or basil leaves = a few, preferably fresh
Lime or lemon = 1, cut in half

Optional:
Bitter melon= use a whole bitter melon, lightly scrape the surface,
then slice it like a cucumber. Use only 2-4 small pieces, because it
is quite bitter. Save the rest for later use. You can get fresh bitter
melon from an Indian-Pakistani or a Chinese-Japanese grocery
store.
Daikon Radish = 1/2, peeled, chopped
Arugula = 1 cup, chopped
Cumin seeds = 1 teaspoon
Clove powder = 1/2 teaspoon
Black pepper= 2 teaspoons OR Cayenne pepper = 1 teaspoon

In a large pot, add 2 tablespoons of olive oil and 4-5 cups
of water. Then add both types of lentils, turmeric, cinnamon stick,
celery, fenugreek seeds, bitter melon pieces and salt. Cook on low
heat for about 45 minutes, stirring occasionally.

Add spinach, Daikon radish, arugula and cook for another 10 minutes.

In the meantime, use a small pan to make what is called *Tarka* in Indian cooking. Add 8 tablespoons of olive oil, chopped onions and garlic to the pan. Cook on low heat for 10 minutes, stirring frequently, until onions start to turn brown. *Tarka* is ready. Pour it into the pot of lentils. Stir well.

In the end, add a few cilantro or oregano or basil leaves . Squeeze and add lime or lemon. Add vinegar. Mix well. Let it sit for about 10-15 minutes before serving.

Optional:
In the beginning, add black pepper OR cayenne pepper, clove powder, fenugreek seeds and cumin seeds.

Add cumin seeds along with onions while making Tarka.

Tip:
Serve it with a salad dish and plain yogurt on the side. Avoid rice or any bread.

MEAT DISHES

Chicken-Vegetable Soup

Cooking time = About 30 minutes

Ingredients:

Chicken breast= 1 Lbs., cut into pieces
Spinach = 1 bunch (approximately 1 cups), washed
Sweat Peas = 1/2 cup
Zucchini = 1, sliced
Celery Stick = 2, cut into small pieces
Yogurt, plain = 1 tablespoon
Olive oil = 2 tablespoons
Balsamic Vinegar = 1/2 teaspoon
Turmeric = 1/2 teaspoon
Black pepper, ground = 1/2 teaspoon
Sea-Salt = 1/2 teaspoon (or regular salt)
Cinnamon = 1 stick
Garlic = 2 cloves, sliced
Onions = 1 medium size, chopped
Ginger root, fresh = about 1/2 inch square, chopped

Optional:

Cayenne pepper = 1/2 teaspoon
Paprika = 1/2 to 2 teaspoons per your taste
Arugula = 1/2 cup
Collard green = chopped, 1/2 cup
Turnip leaves = Chopped, 1/2 cup

In a large pot, add olive oil, onions, celery, salt, garlic, ginger, cinnamon stick, and turn heat to low. Keep stirring frequently.

After about 5 minutes, add chicken, and yogurt, turmeric, Balsamic vinegar and black pepper.

Optional: Add Cayenne pepper OR paprika

Mix in well. Let it cook for about 5-10 minutes, stirring frequently until chicken turns white.

Then, add 4 cups of water. Also add spinach and sweet peas.

Optional : Add other leaves (Arugula, Collard green or Turnip leaves)

Cover and let it cook for another 15 minutes, on low heat.

Add Zucchini and, let it cook another 2 - 3 minutes.

Chicken Nuggets
(Kids and teenagers love them)

Cooking Time = About 30 - 45 minutes

Ingredients:

Chicken = Boneless, preferably breast, about 1 Lb., cut into pieces about 2 x 1 inches
Yogurt = 3 tablespoons
Olive oil = 2 tablespoon
Lime or lemon = 1, cut in half
Apple cider vinegar = 1 teaspoon
Mustard, Dijon = 1 teaspoon
Garlic powder = 1 tablespoon
Sea-Salt = 1 teaspoon

Optional:

Cayenne pepper or black pepper = 1/2 teaspoon

In a large pan, add olive oil, yogurt, apple cider vinegar, Dijon mustard, garlic powder and salt. Squeeze lime or lemon into it. Add 3 tablespoons of water. Mix well.

Optional: Sprinkle Cayenne pepper or black pepper and mix well.

Marinate chicken nuggets in the pan for about 15 - 30 minutes.

Place the pan on <u>medium</u> heat. Stir frequently. Cook nuggets on medium heat for about 5 - 10 minutes, until all yogurt is dried out. Lower the heat and cook for another 5 minutes, until nuggets have turned golden in parts.

Chicken - Bell Pepper

Cooking Time = About 15 minutes

Ingredients:

Chicken = 2 chicken breasts, cut into chunks or 4 drumsticks
Bell pepper = 2 medium, any color, preferably red, cut into chunks
Olive oil = 4 tablespoons
Celery: 1 stick, sliced into small pieces
Onion = 2 medium, chopped
Garlic = 2 cloves, sliced
Tomatoes = 4, chopped
Mustard, Dijon (or yellow) = small amount
Vinegar = Any type, preferably Balsamic, 1 teaspoon
Cilantro or Basil or Mint leaves

Optional:
Sea- Salt = 1 teaspoon
Cumin seeds (or powder) or Caraway seeds = 1/2 teaspoon
Turmeric powder = 1/2 teaspoon
Black pepper = 1 teaspoon OR Cayenne pepper = 1/2 teaspoon

Add olive oil onion, garlic and celery in a big pot and place it on low heat. Cook for about 5 minutes, stirring frequently, until the onions have turned yellowish brown.

Then add chicken chunks, mustard and tomatoes. Turn the heat to medium and cook for about 5 minutes, stirring frequently. Turn heat to low. Add bell pepper. Cook uncovered for about 3 -5 minutes. Add cilantro, basil or mint leaves.

Optional:
In the beginning, add salt, turmeric powder, cumin (or caraway seeds), black pepper OR cayenne pepper.

Ground Turkey or Ground Chicken - Bell Pepper

Cooking Time = About 25 minutes

Ingredients:

Ground turkey (or chicken) = 1 pound
Bell pepper = 2 medium, any color, preferably red, cut into chunks
Olive oil = 2 tablespoons
Onion = 1 medium, chopped
Garlic = 2 or 3 cloves, sliced
Tomatoes = 2 medium, chopped
Sea-Salt = ½ teaspoon (to taste)
Turmeric powder = ¼ teaspoon
Basil leaves, preferably fresh = 8-10 OR 1 teaspoon dried

Optional:

Cumin (or Caraway seeds) = 1/2 teaspoon
Cayenne pepper or black pepper = 1/2 teaspoon

Use a medium size pot. Sauté onion and garlic in olive oil until translucent. Add 1/4 cup of water, turmeric powder and tomatoes, and cover. Cook for another 5 minutes on low heat.

Then, add ground turkey or chicken. Break up meat so that it is in small pieces. Cook until pink is gone, which takes about 5 - 10 minutes.

Add bell pepper. Cook on low heat, uncovered, for about 3 - 5 minutes. Add basil leaves in the end.

Optional:
In the beginning, add cumin (or caraway seeds), black pepper OR cayenne pepper after adding water.

Ground Turkey or Ground Chicken - Zucchini

Cooking Time = About 25 minutes

Ingredients:

Ground turkey (or chicken) = 1 pound
Zucchini = 2 medium, unpeeled, sliced
Olive oil = 2 tablespoons
Onion = 1 medium, chopped
Garlic = 2 or 3 cloves, sliced
Tomatoes = 2 medium, chopped
Clove powder = 1/2 teaspoon
Sea-Salt = ½ teaspoon (to taste)
Turmeric = ¼ teaspoon
Basil OR Oregano leaves = Fresh, 8-10 OR dried = 1 teaspoon

Optional:

Cumin (or Caraway seeds) = 1/2 teaspoon
Cayenne pepper or black pepper = 1/2 teaspoon

Use a medium size pot. Sauté onion and garlic in olive oil until translucent. Add 1/4 cup of water, turmeric powder and tomatoes, and cover. Cook for another 5 minutes on low heat.

Then, add ground turkey or chicken. Break up meat so that it is in small pieces. Cook until pink is gone, which takes about 5 - 10 minutes.

Add zucchini and cloves. Cook on low heat, uncovered, for about 3 -5 minutes. Add oregano or basil leaves.

Optional:
In the beginning, add cumin (or caraway seeds), black pepper OR cayenne pepper after adding water.

Ground Turkey or Ground Chicken - Green Beans

Cooking Time = About 25 minutes

Ingredients:

Ground turkey (or chicken) = 1 pound
Green beans = 20
Olive oil = 2 tablespoons
Onion = 1 medium, chopped
Garlic = 2 or 3 cloves, sliced
Tomatoes = 2 medium, chopped
Dijon mustard = 1 tablespoon
Sea-Salt = ½ teaspoon (to taste)
Turmeric = ¼ teaspoon
Cilantro, Basil or Oregano leaves = fresh 8-10 or dried, 1
    teaspoon

Optional:

Cumin (or Caraway seeds) = 1/2 teaspoon
Cayenne pepper or black pepper = 1/2 teaspoon

Use a medium size pot. Sauté onion and garlic in olive oil until translucent. Add 1/4 cup of water, turmeric powder and tomatoes, and cover. Cook for another 5 minutes on low heat.

Then, add ground turkey or chicken. Break up meat so that it is in small pieces. Cook until pink is gone, which takes about 5 - 10 minutes. Add green beans and Dijon mustard. Cook on low heat, uncovered, for about 5 - 10 minutes. In the end, add cilantro or oregano or basil leaves.

Optional:
In the beginning, add cumin (or caraway seeds), black pepper OR cayenne pepper after adding water.

Ground Turkey or Ground Chicken - Eggplant

Cooking Time = About 25 minutes

Ingredients:

Ground turkey (or chicken) = 1 pound
Eggplant = 2, preferably Japanese or Chinese, sliced
Yogurt = 2 tablespoons
Olive oil = 2 tablespoons
Onion = 1 medium, chopped
Garlic = 2 or 3 cloves, sliced
Tomatoes = 2 medium, chopped
Sea-Salt = ½ teaspoon (to taste)
Turmeric = ¼ teaspoon
Basil leaves = Preferably fresh 8-10 or dried, 1 teaspoon
Pine nuts = a handful

Optional:

Cumin (or Caraway seeds) = 1/2 teaspoon
Cayenne pepper or black pepper = 1/2 teaspoon

Use a medium size pot. Sauté onion and garlic in olive oil until translucent. Add 1/4 cup of water, turmeric powder and tomatoes, and cover. Cook for another 5 minutes on low heat.

Then, add ground turkey or chicken. Break up meat so that it is in small pieces. Cook until pink is gone, which takes about 5 - 10 minutes. Add eggplant and yogurt. Cook on low heat, covered, for about 10 minutes. In the end, add pine nuts and basil leaves.

Optional:
In the beginning, add cumin (or caraway seeds), black pepper OR cayenne pepper after adding water.

Ground Turkey or Ground Chicken - Spinach

Cooking Time = About 25 minutes

Ingredients:

Ground turkey (or chicken) = 1 pound
Spinach = 4-5 handfuls
Yogurt = 2 tablespoons
Olive oil = 2 tablespoons
Onion = 1 medium, chopped
Garlic = 2 or 3 cloves, sliced
Tomatoes = 2 medium, sliced
Sea-Salt = ½ teaspoon (to taste)
Turmeric = ¼ teaspoon
Cilantro or oregano leaves = Preferably fresh 8-10 OR dried, teaspoon dried

Optional:

Cumin (or Caraway seeds) = 1/2 teaspoon
Cayenne pepper or black pepper = 1/2 teaspoon

Use a medium size pot. Sauté onion and garlic in olive oil until translucent. Add 1/4 cup of water, turmeric powder and tomatoes, and cover. Cook for another 5 minutes on low heat.

Then, add ground turkey or chicken. Break up meat so that it is in small pieces. Cook until pink is gone, which takes about 5 - 10 minutes. Add spinach and yogurt. Cook on low heat, uncovered, for about 10 minutes. In the end, add cilantro or oregano leaves.

Optional:
In the beginning, add cumin (or caraway seeds), black pepper OR cayenne pepper after adding water.

Ground Turkey or Ground Chicken - Carrots

Cooking Time = About 25 minutes

Ingredients:

Ground turkey (or chicken) = 1 pound
Carrots= 3 medium sized, peeled, chopped
Celery = 1 stick, chopped
Olive oil = 2 tablespoons
Onion = 1 medium, chopped
Garlic = 2 or 3 cloves, sliced
Tomatoes = 2 medium , sliced
Sea-Salt = ½ teaspoon (to taste)
Cinnamon = ¼ teaspoon
Basil leaves = Preferably fresh or 1 teaspoon dried

Optional:

Cumin (or Caraway seeds) = 1/2 teaspoon
Cayenne pepper or black pepper = 1/2 teaspoon

Use a medium size pot. Sauté onion and garlic in olive oil until translucent. Add 1/4 cup of water, celery and tomatoes, and cover. Cook for another 5 minutes on low heat.

Then, add ground turkey or chicken. Break up meat so that it is in small pieces. Cook until pink is gone, which takes about 5 - 10 minutes. Add carrots. Cook on low heat, uncovered, for about 3 -5 minutes. In the end, add basil leaves.

Optional:
In the beginning, add cumin (or caraway seeds), black pepper OR cayenne pepper after adding water.

Ground Turkey or Ground Chicken - Sweet Peas

Cooking Time = About 25 minutes

Ingredients:

Ground turkey (or chicken) = 1 pound
Sweet peas = 1 cup
Olive oil = 2 tablespoons
Onion = 1 medium, chopped
Garlic = 2 or 3 cloves, sliced
Tomatoes = 2 , sliced
Sea-Salt = ½ teaspoon (to taste)
Turmeric = ¼ teaspoon
Basil and Oregano leaves = Preferably fresh 8-10 or dried, 1
teaspoon

Optional:

Cumin (or Caraway seeds) = 1/2 teaspoon
Cayenne pepper or black pepper = 1/2 teaspoon

      Use a medium size pot. Sauté onion and garlic in olive oil until translucent. Add 1/4 cup of water, turmeric powder and tomatoes, and cover. Cook for another 5 minutes on low heat.

      Then, add ground turkey or chicken. Break up meat so that it is in small pieces. Cook until pink is gone, which takes about 5 - 10 minutes. Add sweet peas. Cook on low heat, uncovered, for about 3 -5 minutes. In the end, add basil and oregano leaves.

Optional:
In the beginning, add cumin (or caraway seeds), black pepper OR cayenne pepper after adding water.

Ground Turkey or Ground Chicken - Cauliflower

Cooking Time = About 25 minutes

Ingredients:

Ground turkey (or chicken) = 1 pound
Cauliflower = 1 cauliflower head, chopped into 10 -12 small pieces
Ginger root = A piece about 2 inches x 1 inch. Peeled and sliced
Yogurt = 2 tablespoons
Celery = 1 stick, chopped
Olive oil = 2 tablespoons
Onion = 1 medium, chopped
Garlic = 2 or 3 cloves, sliced
Tomatoes = 2 , sliced
Sea-Salt = ½ teaspoon (to taste)
Turmeric = ¼ teaspoon
Cilantro or Basil or Mint leaves = Preferably fresh 8-10 or dried, 1 teaspoon

Optional:

Cumin (or Caraway seeds) = 1/2 teaspoon
Cayenne pepper or black pepper = 1/2 teaspoon

Use a medium size pot. Sauté onion and garlic in olive oil until translucent. Add 1/4 cup of water, turmeric powder, ginger, celery and tomatoes, and cover. Cook for another 5 minutes on low heat.

Then, add ground turkey or chicken. Break up meat so that it is in small pieces. Cook until pink is gone, which takes about 5 - 10 minutes. Add cauliflower and yogurt. Cook on low heat, covered, for about 15 minutes, stirring sparingly. In the end, add cilantro or basil or mint leaves.

Optional:
In the beginning, add cumin (or caraway seeds), black pepper OR cayenne pepper after adding water.

Beef or Lamb - Cauliflower - Bell Pepper

Cooking Time = About 35 minutes

Ingredients:

Beef or Lamb for Stew = 1 Lbs., cut into chunks
Cauliflower = 1 of the whole cauliflower head, chopped into 10 -12 small pieces
Bell pepper = 2 medium, any color, preferably red, cut into chunks
Yogurt = 2 tablespoons
Olive oil = 6 tablespoons
Celery = 1 stalk, sliced into small pieces
Onion = 1 medium, chopped
Garlic = 2 clove, sliced
Ginger root = A piece about 2 inches x 1 inch. Peeled and sliced
Mustard, Dijon, (or regular, yellow) = small amount
Vinegar = Any type, preferably Balsamic, 1 teaspoon
Sea-Salt = 1 teaspoon
Cumin seeds (or powder) or Caraway seeds = 1/2 teaspoon
Turmeric powder = 1/2 teaspoon
Cilantro OR Basil Or Mint leaves = Fresh 8-10 OR dried, 1 teaspoon

Optional:

Black pepper = 1 teaspoon OR Cayenne pepper = 1/2 teaspoon

In a big pot on low heat, add olive oil and warm. Add onion, ginger, cumin seeds and salt. Cook for about 5 minutes, stirring frequently, until the onions have turned yellowish brown. Add beef chunks, mustard, turmeric powder, vinegar and yogurt.

Optional: Add black pepper OR cayenne pepper.

Turn the heat to medium and cook for about 5 minutes, stirring frequently.

Turn heat to low. Add cauliflower, tomatoes, garlic and celery. Cover and let it cook for about 30 minutes. Check only once or twice to make sure water is still there. Avoid frequent uncovering. It will reduce the amount of steam, which is cooking the beef and cauliflower.

Uncover. Add bell pepper. Cook uncovered for about 5 minutes. Cook longer to dry it up, if you wish. In the end, add cilantro or mint or basil leaves. Mix well.

Beef or Lamb - Spinach

Cooking Time = About 45 minutes

Ingredients:

Beef or Lamb for Stew = 1 Lbs., cut into chunks
Spinach = about 4 handfuls
Yogurt = 2 tablespoons
Olive oil = 8-10 tablespoons
Butter = 1/2 stick
Celery = 1 stalk, chopped
Onion = 2, medium, chopped
Garlic = 2 clove, sliced
Ginger root = A piece about 2 inches x 1 inch. Peeled and sliced
Mustard = Dijon or regular yellow, small amount
Vinegar = Any type, preferably Balsamic, 1 teaspoon
Sea-Salt = 1 teaspoon
Turmeric powder = 1/2 teaspoon
Cilantro or Basil or Mint leaves = 8-10 fresh OR dried, 1 teaspoon

Optional:

Mustard greens = 4 handfuls, chopped
Collard greens = 2 handfuls
Black pepper = 1 teaspoon OR Cayenne pepper = 1/2 teaspoon.

In a medium size pot on low heat, add 4 tablespoons of olive oil, one chopped onion, ginger and salt. Cook for about 5 minutes, stirring frequently until the onions have turned yellowish brown. Add beef or lamb chunks, mustard, turmeric powder, vinegar and yogurt.

Optional: Add black pepper, OR cayenne pepper.

Turn the heat to medium and cook for about 5 minutes, stirring frequently.

In a separate large pot, add 4 - 6 tablespoons of olive oil, garlic, one chopped onion and spinach.

<u>Optional</u>: Add mustard greens and collard greens.

Cover and let it cook for about 30 minutes. Then, pour it into a blender and grind on low until all leaves are well ground. Pour it back into the large pot.

Empty beef or lamb chunks mixture into this large pot. Mix well. Add butter. Cook for another 15 - 20 minutes on low heat, uncovered, till it is not runny any more.

In the end, add cilantro or mint or basil leaves. Mix well.

Juicy Steak

Ingredients:

Steak = Two approx. 12 ounce New York or Filet Mignon cuts
Yogurt = 3 tablespoons
Olive oil = 6 tablespoons
Bell pepper = 1/2, preferable red, chopped
Vinegar = 1 tablespoon
Mustard, Dijon = 2 tablespoons
Garlic powder = 1 tablespoon
Garlic, fresh = 1 clove, peeled and sliced
Lime (or Lemon) = 1, halved
Sea-Salt = 1 teaspoon
Onion = 1 small, chopped
Tomatoes = 2 medium, chopped
Basil leaves, fresh = 1 cup
Black olives = 10, halved
Capers = 2 tablespoons
Mushrooms = 4-5 white mushrooms, sliced
Cranberries = a handful

Optional:

Pine nuts = a handful
Black Pepper = 1 teaspoon or Cayenne pepper = 1/2 teaspoon

Step 1

Marinate steaks in a pan: Add 1 tablespoon olive oil, 1 tablespoon yogurt, 1 tablespoon Dijon mustard, vinegar, garlic powder and 1 teaspoon of salt. Squeeze and add lime (or lemon).

Optional: Add black pepper or cayenne pepper. Mix well.

Place Steaks in this marinate mixture. Cover well with the marinate mixture by flipping them over several times. Let sit for about 30 - 60 minutes.

Step 2

Make your own <u>pesto</u>: Add basil leaves, 2 tablespoons of water, 2 tablespoons of olive oil, red bell pepper, 1 teaspoon of salt and garlic powder into a blender.

<u>Optional</u>: Add a handful of pine nuts.

Turn the blender on for a minute or so, until the basil leaves are ground into a paste. Empty your pesto into a container.

Step 3

Make your own <u>sauce</u>: In a small pan on low heat, add 3 tablespoons olive oil, onions and sliced garlic. Cook for about 5 minutes. Stir frequently. Onions should be translucent, yellowish but not brown. Then, add 1/2 cup water, 2 tablespoons yogurt, 1 tablespoon Dijon mustard, tomatoes and 1 tablespoon homemade pesto. Mix well. Cook on low heat for another 25-30 minutes, stirring frequently, until it is paste like. In the end, add cranberries, capers, black olives and mushrooms. Your own sauce is now ready.

Step 4

Broil steaks in an Oven for about 5-10 minutes each side, depending upon your taste of rare, medium or well done.

Step 5

Transfer steaks onto a dish. Cover them with your already cooked sauce. Let sit for about 5 minutes before serving.

Tip: Serve it with Salad No. 2 or 3. Great for lunch or dinner.

Zesty Lamb Chops

Ingredients:

Lamb chops = 8
Yogurt = 4 tablespoons
Olive oil = 2 tablespoons
Garlic powder = 1 teaspoon
Ginger powder= 1 teaspoon
Cumin Powder = 1/2 teaspoon
Coriander powder = 1/2 teaspoon
Clove powder = 1/2 teaspoon
Basil dried leaves = 1 teaspoon
Oregano dried leaves = 1 teaspoon
Mustard, Dijon or regular yellow = small amount
Apple cider vinegar = 1 teaspoon

Optional:

Black pepper = 1 teaspoon OR Cayenne pepper = 1/2 teaspoon

In a large pan, add olive oil, yogurt, ginger, garlic, cumin, coriander, clove powder, basil leaves, oregano leaves, Dijon mustard and vinegar. Add a couple of tablespoons of water. Mix well to form a paste.

Optional: Add black pepper OR cayenne pepper.

Place lamb chops in the pan. Holding them by their bony stick, cover them well with the paste on each side. Cover them and marinate for 1 - 2 hours.

Place the pan on a stove, uncovered, at medium to high heat for 5 minutes. Then, lower the heat and cook for another 5-10 minutes, depending upon your taste - rare, medium or well done.

Tip: Use a side dish of one of the salads in this book.

Zesty Lamb Chops - Broccoli - Cauliflower - Eggplant

Ingredients:

Lamb chops, cooked according to the previous recipe
Broccoli = 4 - 6 florets
Cauliflower = 4 - 6 florets
Eggplant = 2, preferably Japanese or Chinese, sliced
Olive oil = 2 tablespoons
Onion = 1 medium, chopped
Mustard, Dijon = 1 tablespoon
Tomatoes = 2, chopped
Cumin seeds = 1/2 teaspoon
Turmeric = ¼ teaspoon

Optional:

Cayenne pepper or black pepper = 1/2 teaspoon.

In a large pan, add olive oil and 1/2 cup of water. Add broccoli, cauliflower, eggplant, cumin seeds, turmeric and Dijon mustard.

Optional: Add black pepper OR cayenne pepper.

Cover and cook on medium heat. Let it cook for about 10 minutes. Check only once or twice to make sure water is still there. Avoid frequent uncovering. It will reduce the amount of steam, which is cooking the vegetables.

Add onions and tomatoes. Turn the heat to low and cook for about 5 minutes, stirring frequently. In the end, add pre-cooked lamb chops. Cover and let it cook on low heat for 2- 3 minutes.

Zesty Beef Stir Fry

Cooking time = About 15 minutes

Ingredients:

Beef for stir fry = 1/2 to 3/4 Lbs., cut into chunks
Yogurt = 2 Tablespoons
Celery = 1 stalk, sliced into small pieces
Zucchini = 1, medium, peeled and sliced
Carrot = 2, small, peeled and cut into small pieces
Bell Pepper = 1, medium, cut into small pieces
Tomato = 1, medium, chopped
Basil leaves = 5, fresh or 1/2 teaspoonful of dried, crushed leaves
Onion = 1, medium, chopped
Ginger = Fresh, 1 inch X 2 inches, peeled and sliced or 1/2
teaspoon of powdered ginger
Garlic = 1 clove, peeled and sliced
Mustard, yellow = 1/2 tablespoon
Sea-Salt = 1/2 teaspoon
Balsamic vinegar = 1/4 teaspoon
Olive Oil = 2 Tablespoon

Optional:

Yogurt = 2 tablespoons
Cayenne pepper or black pepper = 1/2 teaspoon
Turmeric = ¼ teaspoon
Coriander, ground = 1 teaspoon
Cumin, powder = 1 teaspoon
Cloves, whole = 5

In a medium hot wok, add olive oil, onion, celery, zucchini
and yogurt. After a couple of minutes, add beef. Stir continuously.
After a couple of minutes, add salt, garlic, ginger, vinegar and
mustard.

Optional: Add coriander, cumin, turmeric, cloves and hot cayenne
pepper. Continue to stir.

After about 5 minutes, add 1/2 cup of water. Add carrots and cover. Lower the heat and let it cook for another 5 minutes. Stir periodically.

Then, add bell pepper, tomato and basil leaves. Cook for another 2-3 minutes. Let it cool for a few minutes before serving.

Ground Beef - Sweet Peas - Carrots - Olives

Cooking time = About 25 minutes

Ingredients:

Ground beef = 1 pound
Sweet Peas = 1 cup
Carrots = 3 medium sized, peeled, chopped
Mustard, Dijon = 1/2 tablespoon
Black olives = 15, halved
Celery = 1 stick, chopped
Ginger root = A piece about 2 inches x 1 inch. Peeled and sliced
Olive oil = 3 tablespoons
Onion = 1 medium, chopped
Garlic = 2 or 3 cloves, sliced
Sea-Salt = ½ teaspoon (to taste)
Cilantro or Basil leaves = Preferably fresh 8-10 OR dried, 1
     teaspoon
Yogurt = 2 tablespoons

Optional:

Cayenne pepper or black pepper = 1/2 teaspoon
Turmeric = ¼ teaspoon
Coriander, ground = 1 teaspoon
Cumin, powder = 1 teaspoon

     Add olive oil, onions, celery, ginger, and garlic in a medium size pot. Cook on medium heat for about 5-10 minutes, until onions are translucent and yellowish. Stir frequently.

     Add ground beef. Break up meat so that it is in small pieces. Cook until pink is gone, which takes about 5 minutes. Add yogurt and Dijon mustard and cook for a couple of minutes. Lower the heat, and add sweet peas and carrots.

<u>Optional</u>: Add cayenne pepper or black pepper, turmeric, coriander and cumin at the beginning.

Cook on low heat, uncovered, for about 10 -15 minutes, stirring frequently. In the end, add black olives, cilantro or basil leaves.

Tip: You can make lettuce wraps out of it.

Beef Stew 1

Cooking time = About 100 minutes

Ingredients:

Beef stew meat = 1 pound, cut into chunks
Yogurt, plain = 3 tablespoons
Carrots = 2, medium, peeled and cut into pieces
Turnip = 1, peeled, chopped into small pieces
Celery = 1 stalk, cut into small pieces
Onion = 1 medium, peeled, cut into chunks
Garlic = 2 cloves, peeled, cut into small pieces
Ginger root = 1 small piece about 2 inches x 1 inch, peeled and cut into small pieces
Turmeric powder = 1/4 teaspoon
Coriander powder = 1/4 teaspoon
Cumin powder = 1/4 teaspoon
Paprika = 1/4 teaspoon
Sea-Salt = 1/2 teaspoon.
Balsamic vinegar = 1/4 teaspoon

Rinse Beef stew meat chunks and place them in a large pot. Add Yogurt, Onion, Celery, Turnip, Garlic, Ginger, Turmeric, Coriander, Cumin, Paprika, Salt and about 3 tablespoons of water. Mix well and marinate for about 5 minutes.

Then, cook on high heat. Stir frequently until the meat turns brown, about 5 minutes.

Add 3 cups of hot water. Cover and turn heat to very Low. Let cook for about 30 minutes, stirring periodically.

Add Carrots and let it simmer, covered, for another 60 minutes, stirring occasionally. Then, add Balsamic Vinegar. Stir and let it cool for about 5 minutes before serving.

Beef Stew 2

Cooking time = About 45 minutes

Ingredients:

Beef chunks = 1 - 2 Lbs., cut into chunks
Bell pepper = 1 - 2, cut into chunks
Spinach = 1 bunch (approximately 2 cups), washed
Celery Stick = 2, cut into small pieces
Tomatoes = 4 - 6 medium, cut into chunks
Yogurt, plain = 4 tablespoons
Cloves, whole = 4
Olive oil = 2 tablespoons
Turmeric = 1/2 teaspoon
Sea-Salt = 1/2 teaspoon
Cinnamon = 1 stick
Cumin seeds (or powder) = 1 teaspoon
Coriander ground = 1 teaspoon
Garlic = 2 cloves, sliced
Onions = 2 medium size, chopped
Ginger root, fresh = about 1/2 inch square, chopped

Optional:

Cayenne pepper = 1/2 to 1 teaspoon per your taste
Paprika = 1 to 2 teaspoons per your taste

In a large pot, add about 2-3 tablespoons of water, olive oil, onions, celery, salt, garlic, ginger, turmeric, cinnamon stick, cloves, cumin seeds and coriander powder and turn on heat to medium. Keep stirring frequently.

Optional:

Add Cayenne pepper OR paprika.

After about 5 minutes, add beef and yogurt. Mix in well. Adjust the heat to low and cover. Let it cook for about 30 minutes, stirring frequently.

Then, add spinach and bell pepper. Cover and let it cook for another 10 minutes, stirring frequently.

Add tomatoes, cover and let it cook another 5 minutes, stirring frequently.

* You can use Cayenne pepper if you like it hot OR Paprika which is very mild. You can also add two whole dried cayenne peppers if you like it extra hot.

FISH

White Fish - Pan Fried

Cooking Time = About 15 minutes

Ingredients:

White Fish filets = 2 (about 2/3 Lbs.)
Olive oil = 1 tablespoon
Vinegar = 1/2 teaspoon
Mustard, yellow or Dijon = small amount
Lime (or lemon) = 1, cut in half
Garlic powder = 1 teaspoon
Sea-Salt = 1/2 teaspoon
Basil leaves and Rosemary leaves = a few, preferably fresh

Optional:

Black Pepper = 1 teaspoon OR Cayenne pepper = 1/2 teaspoon

First marinate fish filet: Put olive oil into a large pan. Place fish filets in it, side by side. Squeeze lime (or lemon) on the filets. Then, sprinkle garlic powder.

Optional: Add black pepper OR cayenne pepper.

Then, squeeze mustard directly on the filet. Let it sit for about 5 minutes.

Cook the filets in a pan on medium heat for about 5 minutes. Then, turn the filets over and cook for another 5 minutes or so, depending on the thickness of the filets.

Turn heat off. Sprinkle basil leaves and fresh rosemary leaves over filets.

Trout - Pan Fried

Cooking Time = About 20 minutes

Ingredients:

Trout filets = 2 (about 2/3 Lbs.)
Olive oil = 6 tablespoons
Vinegar = 1 tablespoon
Mustard, Dijon = 1 tablespoon
Garlic powder = 1 tablespoon
Lime (or lemon) = 1, cut in half
Sea-Salt = 1/2 teaspoon
Onion = 1 small, chopped
Tomatoes, cherry = 8-10, halved
Basil leaves, fresh = 1 cup
Garlic, fresh = 1 clove, peeled and sliced
Black olives = 10
Capers = 2 tablespoons

Optional:

Black Pepper = 1 teaspoon OR Cayenne pepper = 1/2 teaspoon

Step 1:

Start out by making your own pesto as follows: Add a cupful of fresh basil leaves, 2 tablespoons of water, 2 tablespoons olive oil, black olives, and fresh garlic slices into a blender. Turn it on for a minute or so, until the basil leaves are ground into a paste. Empty your pesto into a container.

Step 2:

Marinate fish filet: Put one tablespoon of olive oil into a large pan. Add Dijon mustard, vinegar, garlic powder and salt, and squeeze lime (or lemon).

<u>Optional</u>: Add black pepper or cayenne pepper. Mix well.

Place fish filets in this mixture. Cover them well with the marinate mixture, by flipping them over several times. Let them marinate for about 5 minutes.

Step 3:
Make your own <u>sauce</u>: In a small pan, add 3 tablespoons of olive oil, onions and tomatoes, and cook on low heat for about 5 minutes. Stir frequently. You want onions to turn translucent, yellowish but not brown. Then, add one tablespoon of your own pesto. Mix well. Let it cook for another couple of minutes, stirring frequently.

Step 4:
Place fish pan on the stove at medium heat and cook for about 1-2 minutes. Then, turn the filets over and cook for another 1-2 minutes. Turn filets over again and cook for 1-2 minutes. Flip and cook for another 1-2 minutes. Total fish cooking time about 6 minutes.

Step 5:
Transfer fish filets onto a dish. Cover them with your already cooked sauce. Let sit for a couple of minutes before serving.

Tip: Serve it with Salad No. 2 or 3. Great for light dinner.

Salmon - Pan Fried

Cooking Time = About 20 minutes

Ingredients:

Salmon filets = 2 (about 2/3 Lbs.)
Yogurt = 2 tablespoons
Olive oil = 6 tablespoons
Bell pepper = 1/2, preferable red, chopped
Vinegar = 1 tablespoon
Mustard, Dijon = 2 tablespoons
Garlic powder = 2 tablespoons
Garlic, fresh = 1 clove, peeled and sliced
Lime (or lemon) = 1, halved
Sea-Salt = 1 teaspoon
Onion = 1 small, chopped
Tomatoes, cherry = 8-10, halved
Basil leaves, fresh = 1 cup
Black olives = 10, halved
Capers = 2 tablespoons

Optional:

Cranberries = a handful
Pine nuts = a handful
Black Pepper = 1 teaspoon or Cayenne pepper = 1/2 teaspoon

Step 1:

Start out by making your own pesto: Add 1 cup of fresh basil leaves, 2 tablespoons water, 2 tablespoons olive oil, red bell pepper, 1/2 teaspoon of salt and 1 tablespoon of garlic powder into a blender. Optional: Add a handful of pine nuts. Turn the blender on for a minute or so, until the basil leaves are ground into a paste. Empty your pesto into a container.

Step 2:

Marinate fish filet in a pan: Add 1 tablespoon olive oil, 1 tablespoon Dijon mustard, 1 tablespoon vinegar, 1 tablespoon garlic powder and 1/2 teaspoon salt. Squeeze and add lime (or lemon).

Optional: Add black pepper or cayenne pepper. Mix well.

Place fish filets in this marinate mixture and cover them well with the marinate mixture by flipping them over several times. Let sit for about 5 minutes.

Step 3:

Make your own <u>sauce</u>: In a small pan on low heat, add 3 tablespoons olive oil, onions and sliced garlic. Cook for about 5 minutes. Stir frequently. Onions should be translucent, yellowish but not brown. Then, add 1/2 cup of water, yogurt, 1 tablespoon Dijon mustard, tomatoes and your own pesto. Mix well. Let cook on low heat for another 25-30 minutes, stirring frequently, until it is paste like. In the end, add capers and black olives. Your own sauce is now ready.

Step 4:

Cook fish in marinating pan at medium heat for about 2-3 minutes. Then, turn the filets over and cook for another 2 -3 minutes. Turn filets over again and cook for 1-2 minutes each side, one more time. Total fish cooking time about 10 minutes.

Step 5:

Transfer fish filets to a dish. Cover them with your already cooked sauce. Let it sit for a couple of minutes before serving.

Tip: Serve it with Salad No. 2 or 3. Great for light dinner.

Acknowledgements

I gratefully acknowledge Georgie Huntington Zaidi, my editor, who did an extraordinary job of transforming this complex medical book into an easy read. On a personal note, I appreciate her every day for being my soul-mate.

I also sincerely acknowledge the brilliant scientific work of many researchers devoted to the field of Thyroid.

Sarfraz Zaidi, M.D.

www.DoctorZaidi.com

About Dr. Zaidi

Dr. Sarfraz Zaidi is a leading Endocrinologist in the U.S.A. He is a medical expert on Thyroid, Diabetes, Vitamin D and Stress Management. He is the director of the Jamila Diabetes and Endocrine Medical Center in Thousand Oaks, California. He is a former assistant Clinical Professor of Medicine at UCLA.

Books and Articles

Dr. Zaidi is the author of the following books:

"Power of Vitamin D"
"Stress Cure Now"
"Take Charge of Your Diabetes"
"Graves' Disease and Hyperthyroidism"
"Hypothyroidism and Hashimoto's Thyroiditis"
"Stress Management for Teenagers, Parents and Teachers"

In addition, he has authored numerous articles in prestigious medical journals.

Memberships

Dr. Zaidi is a Member of the American Association of Clinical Endocrinologists (AACE). In 1997, Dr. Zaidi was inducted as a Fellow to the American College of Physicians (FACP). In 1999, he was honored to become a Fellow of the American College of Endocrinology (FACE).

Speaker

Dr. Zaidi has been a guest speaker at medical conferences and also frequently gives lectures to the public. He has been interviewed on TV, newspapers and national magazines. Dr. Zaidi is the former director of the Endocrine Clinic at the Olive-View UCLA Medical Center where he taught resident physicians undergoing training in Diabetes and Endocrinology.

Internet

Dr. Zaidi also regularly writes on websites including:

www.OnlineMedinfo.com which provides in-depth knowledge about endocrine disorders such as Thyroid, Vitamin D, Parathyroid, Osteoporosis, Obesity, Pre-Diabetes, Metabolic Syndrome, Menopause, Low Testosterone, Adrenal, Pituitary and more.

www.DiabetesSpecialist.com which is dedicated to providing extensive knowledge to Diabetics.

www.InnerPeaceAndLove.com which is an inspirational website exploring the Mind-Body connection.

He regularly writes on his Blog.
www.onlinemedinfo.com/blog/

He has done educational YouTube videos:

About Vitamin D at **www.youtube.com/user/georgie6988**

About Insulin resistance, diabetes and heart disease at **www.youtube.com/user/TheDiabetesEducation**

His main website: **www.DoctorZaidi.com**

Other Books by Dr. Sarfraz Zaidi, MD

"Graves' Disease And Hyperthyroidism:
What You Must Know Before They Zap Your Thyroid With Radioactive Iodine"

Graves' disease is one of several causes of hyperthyroidism. In "Graves' Disease And Hyperthyroidism," Dr. Zaidi describes how to accurately diagnose and treat Graves' disease as well as other causes of hyperthyroidism.

The medical treatment of Graves' disease has not changed in over 50 years. Sad, but true! The standard, usual treatment with Radioactive iodine is a superficial, myopic approach. It almost always makes you hypothyroid (underactive thyroid state). Then, you need to be on thyroid pills for the rest of your life. In addition, radioactive iodine does not treat the underlying root cause of Graves' disease - autoimmune dysfunction, which continues to smolder and easily erupts into another autoimmune disease. Anti-thyroid drugs do not treat autoimmune dysfunction either. They provide only temporary relief. Often, symptoms return once you stop these drugs. Surgery also does not treat autoimmune dysfunction. It often leads to hypothyroidism as well as many other complications.

Over the last ten years, Dr. Zaidi developed a truly breakthrough approach to get rid of Graves' disease at its roots - autoimmune dysfunction. His patients have benefited tremendously from this approach. Now, its time for you to learn about this ground breaking discovery.

Dr. Zaidi reveals what really causes autoimmune dysfunction that ultimately leads to Graves' disease. His revolutionary treatment strategy consists of five components: His unique Diet for Graves' disease (including original recipes), the link between Vitamin D deficiency and Graves' disease, the connection between Graves' disease and Vitamin B12 deficiency, how Stress causes Graves' disease (and Dr. Zaidi's unique strategy to manage stress) and the judicious use of Anti-Thyroid drugs.

"Stress Cure Now"

In his ground breaking book, Dr. Zaidi describes a truly NEW approach to deal with stress. Dr. Zaidi's strategy to cure stress is based on his personal awakening, in-depth medical knowledge and vast clinical experience. It is simple, direct, original and therefore, profound. He uses logic - the common sense that every human is born with. Using the torch of logic, Dr. Zaidi shows you that the true root cause of stress actually resides inside you, not out there. Therefore, the solution must also resides inside you. In **"Stress Cure Now,"** Dr. Zaidi guides you to see the true root cause of your stress, in its deepest layers. Only then you can get rid of it from its roots, once and for all.

"Take Charge of Your Diabetes"

Insulin resistance is the root cause of diabetes in a majority of people, yet most have not even heard of it. In "Take Charge of Your Diabetes," Dr. Zaidi showcases his ground breaking *5-step strategy* to treat diabetes. Using this approach, learn how Dr. Zaidi's patients achieve excellent control of diabetes, prevent complications of diabetes and above all, do not end up on insulin shots. Learn how those who have been on insulin for years are able to come off insulin.

"Stress Management For Teenagers, Parents And Teachers"

Using logic, Dr. Zaidi cuts through the stress triangle of teenagers, parents and teachers. This original, profound and breakthrough approach is completely different from the usual, customary approaches to manage stress, which simply work as a band-aid, while the volcano underneath continues to smolder. Sooner or later, it erupts through the paper thin layers of these superficial strategies.

Dr. Zaidi guides you step by step on how you can be free of various forms of stress. From peer pressure, to stress from education, to conflict between teenagers, parents and teachers, to anxiety, addictions and ADD, Dr. Zaidi covers every aspect of stress teenagers, parents and teachers experience in their day to day life. Dr. Zaidi's new approach ushers in a new era in psychology, yet this book is such an easy read. It's like talking to a close friend for practical, useful yet honest advice that works.

"Power of Vitamin D"

In this book, Dr. Zaidi provides compelling, comprehensive, yet very practical knowledge about vitamin D deficiency, its health consequences, its diagnosis and treatment (without the risk of toxicity).

All books available at Amazon.com and other online retailers.

www.DoctorZaidi.com

VITAMIN D3

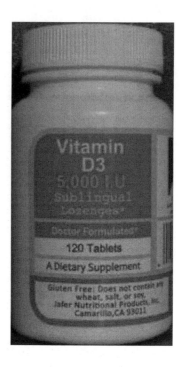

Jafer Nutritional Products,

in collaboration with Dr. Sarfraz Zaidi, MD,

now makes available a high quality Vitamin D3 formula for

Sublingual absorption.

Each tablet contains **5000 IU** of Vitamin D3.

Call (805) 495-7143 or Visit www.DoctorZaidi.com

VITAMIN B12

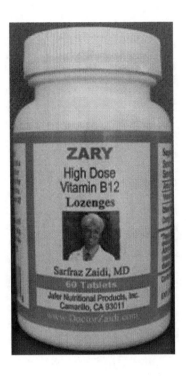

ZARY is a product of Jafer Nutritional Products, which is a vitamin manufacturer of the highest quality.

ZARY is created in collaboration with Dr. Sarfraz Zaidi, MD.

It contains Vitamin B12 in a high dose of 1000 mcg per tablet.

It is formulated as throat lozenges for sublingual absorption.

Call (805) 495-7143 or Visit www.DoctorZaidi.com

GLUPRIDE *Multi*

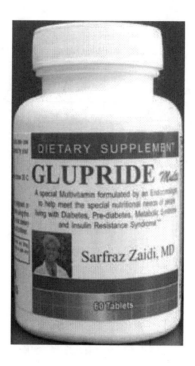

Glupride Multi is a unique vitamin/herbal formula

designed to promote health of people with

Diabetes, Pre-Diabetes and Metabolic Syndrome.

Glupride Multi is created by Sarfraz Zaidi, MD, a respected

Endocrinologist, an expert in the field of Diabetes and Insulin

Resistance Syndrome as well as author of the book,

"Take Charge Of Your Diabetes."

Call (805) 495-7143 or Visit www.DoctorZaidi.com